"This is a wonderful book. It is a ....s system from a unique perspective, explaining posture and the upright position of human beings: including theories that explain the benefits of musculoskeletal therapy from a neurophysiologic perspective."

—Marc D. Braunstein, DO
Past President,
Osteopathic Physicians and Surgeons of California

"Dr. Michael Allen has the ability to educate practitioners of the wonderful benefits of functional neurology in an organized format and easy to comprehend way... I use it every day giving great results."

—Alan Cheng, DC
San Francisco, CA

"This is a very learned and erudite writing. The central theme of *Receptor Based Solutions™* is applied to the reflexes without appearing to hammer the point—a difficult task in any discipline."

—Keith Keen, BA, DipAc, DO, DC, DIBAK
Original developer of techniques related to the neonatal (atypical) display
Sydney, Australia

"You've got me loving how you write and how you've been able to make neurology digestible and understandable for me."

—Susan Walker, BSc, MChiro, DIBAK
Brisbane, Australia

"I have been following Dr. Allen's work over the last twenty plus years, since he published his paper on, 'The Receptor Dependent Nervous System.' It is a work of art to discover all his papers on functional neurology now in one book. I found the addition of clinical cases at the end of each section invaluable. They allow the doctor to put Dr. Allen's ideas into a clinical setting with the kind of patients we all see every day."

—Christopher R. Astill-Smith, D.O., DIBAK
Founder, Epigenetics Limited
Devizes, Wiltshire, England

Receptor Based Solutions™
Functional Neurology Every Doctor Should Know

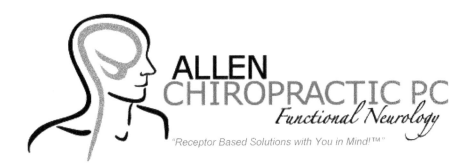

MICHAEL D. ALLEN, DC, NMD, DIBAK, DABCN, FACFN

FUNCTIONAL NEUROLOGIST

www.allenchiropracticpc.com
www.healthbuilders.com

Receptor Based Solutions™
Functional Neurology Every Doctor Should Know

By Michael D. Allen, DC, NMD, DIBAK, DABCN, FACFN

ISBN #: 978-0-9887548-2-9

First Edition

Printed in the United States of America

Disclaimer

The ideas, concepts and opinions expressed in this work are intended to be used for educational purposes only. This book is sold with the understanding that author and publisher are not rendering medical advice of any kind, nor is this book intended to replace medical advice, nor to diagnose, prescribe or treat any disease, condition, illness or injury.

It is imperative that before beginning any diet or exercise program, including any aspect of this work, you receive full medical clearance from a licensed physician.

Author and publisher claim no responsibility to any person or entity for any liability, loss, or damage caused or alleged to be caused directly or indirectly as a result of the use, application or interpretation of the material in this book.

The Food and Drug Administration has not evaluated the statements contained in this book. "Receptor Based Solutions™; Functional Neurology Every Doctor Should Know."

This book is dedicated to all doctors who want to improve their diagnostic and treatment skills, and to all my patients, past, present, and future. To each group, I promise to do my best for you!

Acknowledgements

Writing a functional neurology book can be very intimidating because you want it to be accurate. Doctors and patients depend upon accuracy. But while healing is a science it is also an art, and art is done differently by different people. That is why it is said that doctors have a practice. Every doctor in practice strives to do it right. This text is no exception. I have endeavored to explain these ideas to be best of my ability and to explain it accurately according to my clinical experience.

I wish to thank God for the unique abilities He has given me to understand structure and function. As a junior in high school, I went through every type of test you could ever imagine at the Johnson O'Connor Research Foundation in Los Angeles, California. They reported that I had apparently been blessed with an uncanny ability to visualize structure and they directed me into the field of healthcare. I found my calling.

My practice opened up when I started studying Chiropractic Neurology through the Carrick Institute for Graduate Studies in 1991. Dr. Carrick opened my eyes to the reality that is functional neurology and I have not altered course. Thank you Dr. Carrick.

I would also like to thank my wife, Cindy, for her support while I wrote this second book. I told her I would stop after one, but I could not help myself. She is very understanding.

Two other doctors also have impacted this writing in their own way. My personal friend and colleague, Dr. Keith Keen, has been a pioneer in the understanding of what he refers to as neonatal reflexes. We have had several spirited discussions and his experience has directed much of my understanding. The other doctor is Dr. Susan Walker, who gave me some valuable suggestions in the writing of this text. Thank you to both of you for your input.

Finally, I would like to thank my past, present, and future patients for the opportunity to practice my calling with each of them. I promise to continue to do my best for them.

Stay well!

Contents

SECTION III
Receptor Based Solutions™ for Your Application

Section I

Receptor Based Solutions™ for Your Edification

Introduction to Receptor Based Solutions™

Functional Neurology Every Doctor Should Know

Introduction

Neurology has been one of my favorite subjects since starting my chiropractic journey in 1973—more correctly since I was born. Obviously I did not understand the intricacies of such a wonderful profession in my youngest youth but I did receive a lifelong benefit from it (Figure 1).

Let me explain. You see, I apparently had some hip trouble after I was born that kept me from being a happy sleeper. After a few treatments from our family chiropractor I slept like the proverbial baby. As I grew older, there were times I would go to see my chiropractor just because the treatments felt so good and I understood the idea of prevention; I just wanted to stay well. I remember several treatments when I walked out feeling so well that I thought I could float if I could only raise both my feet from the ground at the same time.

Now more than six decades later I am proud to tell you that I have been a chiropractic patient all my life. I have never had any immunizations, taken any medication or had any surgery aside from dental visits and minor skin issues. I attribute my health to a strong and healthy nervous and immune system that results from regular and natural chiropractic health care.

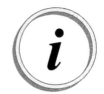

Figure 1: Information is a powerful clinical asset

Looking back, my neighbors were reguarly allowed to eat store bought cookies and candy, drink sodas and the like. Their sandwiches were even made of white bread—they were so lucky! My cookies were few and far between. I was told to eat an apple or a carrot if I were hungry, to drink plenty of water, and my sandwiches were made with whole wheat bread. Imagine!

Well, I thought my neighbors were so special. However, as I reconsider their health they were underweight, regularly sick, and as they have grown and matured their lifestyle choices have not served them well. Although I always thought of my neighbors as being more favored by their parents than I was by mine, it turns out that my parents had the better, more long range plan. I am very thankful for my parent's foresight and the abilities of the chiropractor who took such good care of me and my family in my formative years.

What is Health?

The word "health" indicates a sense of wholeness, wellbeing, soundness of function and being well. It implies a state where the whole body functions optimally without evidence of disease or abnormality.

The World Health Organization has defined health as: "...*a state of complete physical, mental and social well-being and not merely the absence of disease or infirmity.*"

That definition was later modified in part to include the resources of everyday life, but not simply the objective of living.

Most recently, an article in *The Lancet* pointed out that health is not a, "*state of complete physical, mental, and social well-being.*" Neither is it, "*merely the absence of disease or infirmity.*" The article goes on to state that the WHO definitions of health will not do in an era marked by new understandings of disease at molecular, individual, and societal levels.

While these organizations struggle to find a common ground, it is clear that when a person has their health they have both physical and cognitive possession of their innate abilities without hindrance of their activities of daily living.

What makes human brains so unique?

Specific traits set mammals apart from other animals. The same is true with humanity, but humans are unlike animals. The human nervous system is mammalian, but the converse is not true: the mammalian system is not necessarily human. The human nervous system works unlike any other; only the human nervous system is human. A few of the traits that distinguish humans from other species are self-awareness and morality, speech and symbolic cognition, nimble thumbs, upright posture, conscience, sociability, and the capacity to imagine. It is each doctor's responsibility to help each human's brain be as efficient as possible, and that requires that the doctor is constantly learning. Every chapter of these *Receptor Based Solutions™* will address the most appropriate ways to treat the expression of these uniquely human traits from a functional neurology perspective.

For example, achieving upright posture and two-footed gait are two more uniquely human traits and the stimulus for these human expressions is gravity. While gravity pushes things toward the earth, the great majority of the human nervous system is designed to resist gravity's effects resulting in upright, bipedal posture. Further, our bipedal abilities allow movement while using gravity in our favor. It all starts as joints and muscles increase their tone to supply increased influence on the brain and the brain's ability to cause purposeful—and appropriate—movement. With stronger neurological influence comes greater mobility and cognition.

The Receptor-Driven Brain

The human nervous system is optimally driven by receptor input and its motor response is preprogrammed to produce neurotypical—*normal*—human movement patterns that reinforce optimal brain function. Signals cycle with input and response at what seems to be lightning speed. As we will see, these pages—individually and together—are meant to help the doctor consider human performance from a receptor-driven perspective. They focus on the big picture of what neurotypical movement is all about, knitting a better understanding of what it means to be healthy from a neurological perspective since the nervous system is the fundamental feature of all human function.

My friend and AK mentor, Walter Schmitt, DC once said:

"The reason one doctor's technique does not work in another doctor's practice may be that the doctors are employing two very different tools, and mistakenly calling them the same things."

Primitive Reflexes

The more I research and practice with the physiological—also known as neonatal or primitive—reflexes, the more I understand that there is considerable variation between their academic description and their practical application. Therefore, my clinical experience teaches me that the only way to properly apply these reflexes is to stimulate each one of them on every person in order to gain a better understanding of their purposeful neurological status and observe that person's individual response using *functional* manual muscle testing (fMMT). If that person's neurophysiological response to a particular stimulus matches what would be anticipated in a neurotypical human nervous system, then and only then is it fair to say that their reflexes are working according to their originally designed plan. However, if their functional response is anything other than that which is anticipated according to their pre-programmed nature, then that system should always be considered to be pathological because it is a deviation from that which is considered to be normal. Each one of these reflexes should be evaluated and treated according to the person's personal needs, and then reevaluated to see that their performance has been returned to their optimal functional neurological state.

Who Cares?

Who really cares about primitive reflexes? What good are they? Really, why do we need to know about these primitive reflexes and why should a doctor be able to use them properly? What can a doctor really learn about the sensory and motor pathways to the cord and brain and back to the cord again when the foot kicks after the patellar tendon is struck with a reflex hammer? We learned about the patellar reflex in school, right?

A reflex may be defined as an immediate and involuntary response to a stimulus. It is a fast response to a change in the body's internal or external environment in an attempt to maintain balance and stability; i.e., homeostasis.

Most reflexes are protective. They are designed so we can respond to a stimulus faster than we can think. For example, several reflexes keep us upright and others pull us away from pain. Properly working reflexes keep us standing tall and safe.

"Primitive reflexes" (aka infant, infantile, developmental, and/or newborn reflexes) develop *in utero* and are considered by most authors to only persist from a few months to a few years after birth and then they are said to be "extinguished"; they apparently disappear. This idea has always intrigued me because if the primitive reflexes are only found in the very young and then these kids outgrow them, why should we study them? Primitive reflexes tell us of an infant's or toddler's neurological status, but what about after this phase of development when, as other authors have suggested, they are "extinguished?" These same authors go on to say that if and when these reflexes ever return (and this is another issue that will be discussed as we proceed) it is because of some pathology like a stroke, dementia or some other chronic degenerative condition that is unfixable anyway. As we shall discover, many of these dysfunctional reflex expressions can be returned to their normal physiological display.

My good friend, Keith Keen, BA, DipAc, DO, DC, DIBAK, from Sydney, Australia originally developed and subsequently refined many techniques related to the neonatal (atypical) display of these primitive reflexes. Dr. Keen believes that, "Changes in indicators within our own field of expertise do not necessarily mean that there is any change in the patient's function or interaction with environment" so his approach is based upon pre and post correction assessment of the patient by professionals in other fields whose special skill is to assess and quantify neonatal reflexes, behavior, sensory, sensorimotor or learning proficiency.

Dr. Keen goes on to state that, "Primitive reflexes involve automatic and stereotyped movements, respiration, autonomic, and glandular responses which are executed *without cortical involvement.*

Further, "The reflexes anatomically and neurologically stay for the remainder of our life. But for mature voluntarily directed responses to take place, the neonatal display of the reflexes must be integrated or controlled by higher centers." Moreover, Dr. Keen teaches that, "It is the *neonatal display* of these brainstem reflexes continuing after normal time of integration that causes the problems in behavior, perception, learning, hormonal function, etc. ..."

Finally, Dr. Keen concludes that the inappropriate integration of these primitive reflexes can disturb some or all of the functions of higher centers, which include:

Gross motor coordination	Fine motor coordination
Vestibular integration	Auditory perception and integration
Visual function	Cognition and expression
Lateral integration	Social and individual behavior
The development of succeeding primitive and postural reflexes	

Another good friend and colleague of Dr. Keen's, the late James Blumenthal, DC, DACBN, FACFN, wrote of these primitive reflexes:

"If the neonatal reflexes [reappear,] (not properly integrated), they can disturb some or all of the functions of the higher centers, including balance, normal body movements, gross and fine motor control, structural problems, vision, hormonal problems, social cueing, emotional and academic development, anxiety, panic attacks, autistic and attention deficit spectrum symptoms, etc."

The primitive reflexes have been well known to clinicians for decades, yet it appears to be little known that each of these reflexes eventually fits into the background of the human neurological framework. In reality, there is a difference between a dysfunctional primitive reflex display and a retained primitive reflex. It is this author's clinical experience that the normal perseverance and neurological involvement of these primitive reflexes is necessary no matter the person's age. These reflexes should *always* be retained but they should not display pathologically. It is both the primitive reflex's normal and abnormal display that should be clinically important to every doctor. Read that again. It is only when the functionally integrated primitive reflexes display themselves in an *abnormal* manner that there is clinical significance.

Ambiguity Resolved

Let us unpack what has been discussed so far so we can understand this functional reflex idea a bit better. Despite their known characteristics, there are many different thoughts regarding the resilience of these primitive reflexes.

Developmental reflexes seem to arise at various points during intrauterine life and are regularly assessed in pediatric patients to determine a child's level of maturity and if that child is potentially experiencing any delays. Further, it has been taught that primitive reflexes are present in infancy and that they last for a few months to a few years when they eventually disappear as the young brain matures, and that they may reappear at some future point due to various pathologies that disrupt the normal cortical inhibitory pathways. Moreover, the common medical literature generally teaches that the reappearance of these same reflexes after the first year or two of life is always a pathological finding and if they are discovered in an adult it can be attributed to fatigue, or effort, or following central nervous system (CNS) damage. Much of this literature, however, is mainly based upon observations, untested in functional reality. These observations are an exploration of neurological function, but the explorers clearly exhibit an inability to evaluate the reason for some of their own suppositions due to clear biases that others have previously theorized and perpetuated in literature. Their explanations persist through repetition, but as we shall see their literature may not be consistent with clinical practice and independent assessment of results. It is the purpose of these *Receptor Based Solutions*™ to teach the quantifiable approaches to keeping these pathologies from gaining a foothold and prevent—or at least slow—the degenerative changes that lead to the signs and symptoms of neurological disease.

We have clinically found that the interruptions of the cortical inhibitory pathways are most likely secondary to *deafferentation* (the reduction of sensory input), which leads to various frontal release signs; a functional fragmentation of the frontal integrity that is considered to be the seat of humanity. The point being that these dysfunctional primitive reflex findings can be clinically present without frank pathology. The disruptions commonly present themselves in the presence of deafferentation secondary to some breakdown of central integration. But since the medical literature suggests that these reflexes are quickly extinguished, who really looks for them after childhood or before frank degeneration sets in? We do. That is what *Receptor Based Solutions*™ is all about!

21

There is a difference between a reflex's improper integration and its pathological reappearance in later life. And in many cases, fixing the integration problems when they first appear can prevent their pathological progression. Let me say that again: examining every patient's primitive reflex response and returning any dysfunction to its anticipated and preprogrammed display has a very high probability of contributing to a person's healthier neurological experience and life.

A physiological reflex *should always* reappear according to its predesignation every time it is challenged with fMMT techniques and that display is always considered neurotypical. The foregoing and persistent operative misconception that a primitive reflex's return means that the patient has some condition that has upset the certainty or stability of the nervous system is the whole reason for writing *Receptor Based Solutions™*. A neurotypical response is fundamental to the original human program.

We know what to anticipate with each stimulus so we should expect that display every time a particular system is challenged. For example, each time a person turns his or her head one way or the other, or has a tendon stimulated, or their foot stroked, or their hand stroked, or their back scratched there should always be the anticipated display; there should be an anticipated and preprogrammed responsive movement. Any movement other than that which is anticipated is always pathological and must be addressed in order to reestablish normal human behavior.

Therefore, a pathological response is actually any reflex display other than that which has been fundamentally programmed. This erroneous display will not happen in a neurotypical person, so any neurological instability needs treatment to return the patient to their proper neurological display and physiology. As a result of their flawed physiological display, dysfunctional reflexes have a very high probability of being involved in symptoms unique to that person's physiological instability.

The Perception of Reality

What happens if someone's brain becomes sick? How would you know if your brain, or someone else's brain, were sick? Would it hurt? Among several interesting thoughts, F. Matthais Alexander, who founded the Alexander Technique is quoted to have said, "The stupidity of letting children go wrong is that once they go wrong their right is wrong; therefore, the more they try to be right, the more they go wrong." I believe he is exactly correct, and *Receptor Based Solutions™* will examine this idea further.

Our brains are designed for health and give us access to our outside world. They receive environmental input and provide us with the response that is consistent with what we perceived, but too often the inside environment and outside world cause these reflexes to default to sickness. Sometimes our perception and/or our response to that perception is inconsistent with reality and that sets up neurological confusion otherwise known as a mismatch or a timing error. Unless these timing errors are either realized by the person—which, by definition they cannot be because one cannot perceive what they cannot perceive—or found during examination, they become a fundamental part of the dysfunctional neurological matrix and considered to be the person's new normal when in fact they are erroneous. How can a person's nervous system perform according to its preprogrammed nature if its expression is fundamentally inappropriate relative to its original programming? Could a brain that functions in such a way be considered sick? Of course it could.

There are several brain maps that weave functional anatomy and appropriate activity into human majesty. Some of these functional maps tell us where we are in reality while other maps display where we think we are relative to our reality, and many times these maps are contradictory leading to postural imbalances, joint breakdown, pain, injury, and even death from accidental falls.

Fundamental Patterns

What provokes upright posture and what keeps us from falling down?

Upright posture is more than standing up straight, just as walking is more than putting one foot in front of the other to move from place to place. Basic human movement patterns are chalked full of functional reflexes all blended together; they are inborn. Posture is an unconscious practice, and a functional posture is magnificent.

The maturation and integration of elementary movement patterns provides the framework for more mature abilities later in life. For example, a baby cannot do much for themselves right after birth, but once their head extends from their bed their neurological maturation starts in earnest. Extension of the head on the neck appears to be the event that starts the receptor cascade to ignite the nervous system's maturation process.

Actually, the primitive display is not limited to the young. A highly skilled doctor can clinically observe the expressions of primitive reflexes in practice on newborns, infants, toddlers, teens, and mature adults alike. Each level of maturation should express these reflexes neurotypically and the doctor must know how to elicit them properly, and then understand what they are observing in order to return any pathology to normalcy.

The doctor should know each of these normal functional primitive strategies and what it means when they falter. Individually, these reflexes are not useful for localization purposes, but when evaluated as a group—those that are functional versus those that are pathological—they are very helpful to understand the purposeful integrity of the entire neurological display and the functional level to treat in order to return each dysfunctional reflex to normal without disturbing those that are functioning normally.

Dysfunctional Patterns

Large portions of the general population have at least one dysfunctional primitive reflex, and clinical experience has indicated that many people have several. The more dysfunctional reflexes that a person exhibits or the more asymmetrical their display becomes, the more obvious their effects are on the human condition. People with a dysfunctional primitive reflex display can live an apparently normal life without ever exposing their dysfunction to the untrained clinician, but their dysfunction is nonetheless present and has its neurological effect on the more rostral neuraxis. Although a single reflex's dysfunction may not be obvious, it is nonetheless pathological with its own signs and symptoms relative to that person and it needs treatment. As a result, every motor response is influenced by an associated deafferentation, which reinforces the abnormal sensory afferents; sensory conflict often sets up a vicious pathological cycle. Further, as the number of pathological primitive responses rises in any given patient, so does the potential for functional error. In fact, three or more dysfunctional primitive reflex signs often indicate increasingly profound neurological involvement to the point that the dysfunction could mimic a neurological condition known as cerebral palsy. While cerebral palsy is most often caused by an insult to the immature or developing brain—most often before birth—it is nonetheless a profound movement disorder, and that is exactly what we are talking about; movement disorders. Specific reflexes that do not mature as a child grows, and adults who display with atypical neurological performance, often take on an appearance of cerebral palsy, which primarily causes orthopedic impairment and is accompanied by changes in muscle tone, movement coordination and control, reflexes, posture, balance, and fine, gross and oral motor function.

Primitive Reflexes in the Neurological Exam

Primitive reflexes are an integral part of any neurological exam to evaluate cortical (usually frontal lobe) function, especially if there is a suspected brain injury. If the primitive reflexes are not being modulated properly, their expression is more properly called frontal (or cortical) release signs. Clinically, any deafferentation syndrome may present with "cortical release signs" (CRSs), but these are "soft" signs rather than those with more profound pathological involvement that display with "hard" pathology. Research potentially indicates that an atypical primitive reflex display of three or more CRSs may be a possible early warning sign of a more complicated neurological syndrome, including an autistic spectrum disorder (ASD) and other potential learning disabilities secondary to abnormal sensory input, and fixing the sensory input can change the cortical display and help ease these conditions.

It is through these first few stages of life while the cortex is in its most immature state that we depend upon these automatic, instinctual, and involuntary impulses. These primitive reflexes are automatic stereotypic movements directed from the brainstem and require no cortical involvement; they originate within the CNS yet they are individuated and unlinked until they become mature. Actually, primitive reflexes develop in a preprogrammed order and are superlatively integrated into the human neurological design. They are gradually incorporated into the human fabric and modulated by the frontal lobes as a youngster moves through their normal childhood development. This integration is fundamental to the neurotypical interactions of the human nervous system as a whole. We rely on these unripe reflexes for our basic survival and development and grow into them with maturity, but they never leave us. However, any missed aspect of their phased integration can lead to functional errors.

Greatly Exaggerated Reports of Extinction

Primitive reflexes are exhibited by both infants and adults in both neurotypical and erroneous character in response to particular stimuli. For example, any primitive reflex that takes on a display other than that which is according to its original design tends to integrate problems. They can disturb the progression and assimilation of subsequent functional reflexes even disrupting some or all of the functions of higher centers, which as Dr. Keen states includes behavior, learning, the integration of gross or fine movements, and more. And in the words of Alexander, "...the more they try to be right, the more they go wrong." The abnormal display of infantile reflexes can often occur in adults with degenerative and pathological changes (i.e., hard signs) like brain damage and/or stroke. Actually, primitive reflexes can even have an abnormal display without such frank pathology (i.e., soft signs) when the nervous system becomes deafferentated.

The interrelationships of the primitive reflex patterns with mature human performance are fundamental to uniquely human behavior. As our higher cortical centers mature and achieve a higher degree of integration, these primitive reflexes gradually intermingle with the rest of the maturing neurological fabric to create the normal behavior patterns that we call human. The more cohesive cerebral cortex keeps these reflexes intact through its outgoing inhibitory hierarchical influence. However, any subsequent deafferentation of these more rostral centers can lead to CRSs. Said in another way; the cortex begins to "release" its inhibitory influence so the nervous system displays movements that should have otherwise been inhibited. Since these resultant movement patterns are not of a typical human character, they set up a gradual afferent interference pattern that leads to degenerative changes, which slowly chip away at the integrity of the cortical matrix resulting in the signs and symptoms of disease, pain and disintegration.

Sensory Conflict

Did you know that 120 meters per second equals 268 miles per hour, which is 4,716.8 inches per second? This simple fact has to do with functional timing. The speed of the primary afferents (the largest diameter neurons called *proprioceptors*) that arise from muscle spindles and travel to the cord and brain is faster than the length of a football field in one second! And in a person six feet tall, these six feet are traveled practically instantaneously.

In an ideal world, when the incoming signals from one side of the body are consistent with those that arise from the same locations on other side of the body there is balance in the management systems and the motor response has a very high probability of being balanced as well. However, and more realistically, when the sensory input from the two opposite sides of the body are in conflict and their management systems are too broken down to keep up with their discord, timing errors arise that eventually lead to an imbalanced motor response, and that leads to further input errors.

Primary afferents are always sending their signals to the brain, and their input must be spot-on for the brain to respond in kind. If the input is precisely timed, then the output will be according to the original human plan. But if there is conflict anywhere along the sensory input, then the motor response will be likewise flawed, and in some cases the mismatch may preclude any appreciable motor response. Additionally, an accumulative breakdown anywhere along the primary afferentation creates a flaw in the entire homologous neural matrix.

The truth is that no person—child or adult—is free of conflicting sensory input. Everybody has it to some degree. In general, sensory conflict has to do with the brain's inability to rightly modulate body motion in both consistent and inconsistent environments. This is just a truth of our terrestrial existence. Specifically, sensory mismatch is a sign of motor control having gone awry.

Muscle Spasm

In this second example, muscles that lose their ability to produce ATP in a timely manner develop fatigue that allows increased tone, a loss of synchrony for smooth movement—the muscles on one side of a joint relax to accommodate contraction on the other side of that joint—and an eventual spasticity that creeps in slowly. In general, muscles need calcium to contract and ATP to relax. Muscles that function within their capacity have a very high probability of maintaining their ability to make ATP; ATP both encourages and is the result of aerobic endurance. But if a muscle's demands exceeds its capacity—that is, if the muscle cannot produce enough ATP fast enough to promote meaningful work—the muscle can tend toward an increased tone and that asymmetrically modifies its afferents to the cord.

Next, while a person may be able to voluntarily overcome the exaggerated movement synergy (an increased flexor or extensor tone, for example) there is a concomitant reduction in range of motion of the involved joint(s). This could facilitate movement combinations that do not follow preprogrammed synergy patterns, which leads to compensatory complications within the involved joints and an increased probability of injury.

Finally, more difficult movement combinations are developed as basic limb synergies increase their dominance over what were preprogrammed motor acts. All of this adaptation causes concomitant dysfunction within homologous columns, including the cord and brain, leading to further dysfunction in the anterior horn. This represents a change in the central and peripheral neurologic functional stability, i.e., pathology.

Autonomic Concomitants

Each working muscle needs oxygen and fuel, and a way to deliver both of these essential nutrients to the tissues—i.e., there must also be appropriate blood supply. But how does the doctor know if the muscles are getting adequate blood supply? Further, the doctor must know how to evaluate the autonomic concomitants, like blood supply, spinal cord integration and brain performance, etc., and how to best return its dysfunction to its highest level of normalcy.

Without an appropriately maintained autonomic milieu, the human system would be unable to flourish. Further, with each movement comes an associated autonomic response that is essential for structural nourishment and endurance during each movement, but that autonomic response can be either functional or dysfunctional. The doctor should be able to tell the difference. Every doctor should know if a muscle is receiving its requisite needs, and if not, what can be done to best meet these needs.

About 90% of the outflow from the brain (the efferent autonomic drive) has to do with organs and their autonomic controls. Only 10% of the entire cortical outflow goes to muscles. This fact is very important. If the doctor spends more time observing the effects of an fMMT and little to no time monitoring autonomic responses, then he or she may have essentially blinded him or herself to the largest window available to observe functional humanity.

Over time, seemingly benign autonomic problems can lead to the frank signs and symptoms of disease. For example, shoulder girdle troubles can eventually contribute to brain timing errors that set up heart, digestive, vestibular, and/or many other more severe problems, like Parkinson's disease. Did you know that shoulder pain can be the very first symptom a person displays in their windup toward Parkinson's disease?

Primitive Reflexes and Learning

The dysfunctional primitive reflex is a major problem that has the propensity to disrupt the physiological, neurological and biochemical bases of learning and behavior. These are the important issues that need our clinical attention. Every doctor who sees patients with structural problems and movement disorders should know what to anticipate each time a patient moves and how to address the movement problems they find. For example, movements like turning the head one way or the other, flexing and/or extending each leg, rolling over while in bed, standing up from a seated posture, throwing a ball, bending down to pick something up from the floor, or leaning over to brush their teeth all require different patterns of movement, but a reflex's dysfunction can easily put a person's structural instabilities into a degenerative crumple. It is always better to catch these dysfunctional movements before they create more serious problems, and rehabilitate them back to normalcy.

Hierarchical Inhibitory Cascade

In general, the hierarchical controls inherent in the human nervous system (Figure 2) are inhibitory upon the systems below them. This cascade ensures that the lower foci remain under the controls of the segmentally more rostral centers. For example, the cerebral cortex exerts its inhibitory control over the thalamus, and the thalamus has a likewise inhibitory control over the hypothalamus, which has an inhibitory control over the mesencephalon, and it is inhibitory to the reticular centers of the more caudal brainstem. Finally, these brainstem centers have an inhibitory influence over spinal cord centers that facilitate and inhibit certain inborn movement patterns that have their final common effect on the anterior horn of the spinal cord—"the final common pathway". Any disruption of these inhibitory pathways sets up dysfunction

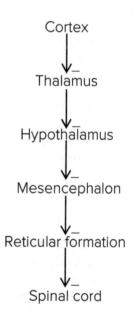

Figure 2: Schematic of hierarchical modulation

that should have otherwise been inhibited. These disruptions are the CRSs that indicated a breakdown of the cerebral cortical modulatory influences with a release of its otherwise purposeful display. Any dysmodulation, mistiming or interruption of the final common pathway will always display an operative musculoskeletal dysfunction, and via the same pathways show the doctor when these modulatory systems have a neurotypical response after treatment.

Consider the foregoing again: Primitive reflexes are present in the newborn and are gradually transformed into a more functional format as the infant's CNS matures. In essence, an infant, toddler's or child's maturation is a steady weaving of these systems into a functional environment that is moored in the frontal lobe of the brain. Any subsequent breakdown of that maturity, which represents an unmooring of these hierarchical patterns—a loss of cortical grouping perhaps secondary to a deafferentation syndrome, or the signs of cortical release—often tends to appear in later life and may be suggestive of—even mimicking—spinal cord injury or damage, diffuse cerebral, subcortical, or bilateral frontal lobe pathology; that is to say that the indications of a CNS disease can be the result of long-standing deafferentation.

Older children and adults with a neurological display inconsistent with that which is considered to be neurotypical (primarily those people thought to have cerebral palsy, but this may also include such conditions as dementia, traumatic lesions, and strokes, including the soft signs of hemisphericity) may permit the escape of these primitive reflexes from their natural cortical controls.

A person's soft signs may appear normal to the untrained eye. Under more extreme conditions—such as during a startle reaction or as the result of some neurological provocation—these reflex dysfunctions often become more obvious. Further, a deafferentation secondary to any movement error can also cause a dysfunction of the cortical inhibitory controls of these reflexes, i.e., it causes the expression of CRSs.

The prevalence of CRSs in schizophrenia, affective disorder, obsessive-compulsive disorder, Alzheimer's disease, vascular dementia, frontotemporal dementia, and other neuropsychiatric disorders like ASD, attention deficit disorder (ADD), attention deficit hyperactivity disorder (ADHD), dyslexia, learning and behavioral difficulties, etc., indicates that these conditions may relate to a breakdown of sensory input consistent with a disturbance in the usual afferent pattern of activity or behavior. This is the definition of deafferentation. Further, the understanding of each dysfunction allows for their use in the clinical management of these patients, including diagnostic assessment, treatment monitoring and prognosis.

A number of issues tend to complicate the interpretation of these CRSs, not the least of which is a lack of specificity and uncertainty over what constitutes an "abnormal" response. As a result, this series of *Receptor Based Solutions*™ will inject new thought based upon clinical and functional neurological reality and create some space between what has clinical relevance and that which has merely been perpetuated by observers.

Eight Important Physiological Reflexes

The key to maintaining each person's uniquely human nervous system lies in the doctor's ability to better understand the preprogrammed human design. Its functional blueprint links the eyes, ears, and spinal muscles with the central neuraxis to maintain upright stability with the extremities while resisting gravity and moving about freely. The deep tendon, tonic neck, flexor withdrawal, crossed cord, Galant, modified Galant, upper Galant (these latter two being uniquely described by this author), and tonic lumbar reflexes each have their own distinct display that should manifest according to their original design when provoked with fMMT procedures. Each of these chapters will discuss each reflex's normal and the abnormal display and go even further to discuss the importance of these reflexes relative to the CRSs. Maintaining an intact cortex and its efferent systems has a very high probability of managing the physiological reflexes that in many cases are controlled by the more rostral neuraxis.

Any movement and/or autonomic response other than that which is according to the original human design is/are clinically pathological and need(s) treatment, and in many cases they are fixable. Once each of these reflex's neurotypical display is restored the nervous system tends to once again function according to its original intent.

Functional Errors

Quiet stance (often referred to as "static balance control," as opposed to those demands involved with perturbations to stance or during locomotion, which require more dynamic forms of control) and gait are important. How does a doctor know if a person's stance and gait contain functional troubles? An observant doctor will have the person move about in various ways and watch their execution of sometimes even the most minor tasks. If a person looks like they stand properly and they are able to walk, is there still trouble? Yes and the doctor should be concerned. Each doctor should know what to look for, how to find it, and how to treat it. And after the issues are treated the patient should be retested and rehabilitated to keep their system working correctly.

Statistics show that the highest incidence of accidental death is related to incidental falls. People fall when their center of gravity exceeds their limits of stability. Once outside their zone of stability, gravity takes over and down they go. Falls happen fast and people hit the ground hard resulting in injuries such as bruises, fractures, concussions, and even death. The doctor should know if a person has a propensity to fall and what to do to keep them from falling. *Receptor Based Solutions™* discusses just such issues with simple tests the doctor can do at each visit with indicators that will help understand how their patients are progressing toward increased stability.

Simple clinical tests such as Romberg test, standing on one foot or the other with eyes open and/or closed, and maintaining upright posture while turning the head through various movements—including the head right and left, and putting the head into flexion and extension—all give valuable clinical understanding about functional neurology. How about just walking, heel to toe walking or walking backwards, the Fakuda test or the pull test? These can all assess stability, individually and together. The eyes are invaluable to elicit paraspinal and/or core dysfunction. Any functional error will be obvious if you know what to look for, and *Receptor Based Solutions™* will help you recognize many of these errors quickly, and teach you how to treat them properly.

Summary

With an aging population, doctors should be searching for movement disorders at every visit. We should be turning errors into accuracies and encouraging a more efficient expression of each patient's uniquely human aspects of posture and gait. *Receptor Based Solutions™* will give the doctor a new clinical perspective all the while giving the patient newfound poise.

Doctors, your patients depend on your abilities to properly diagnose and treat every single one of these functional reflexes and as a result make their brain perform more clearly. If these reflexes break down in later life they may be suggestive of diffuse cerebral, subcortical, or bilateral frontal lobe pathology; the patient may exhibit CRSs.

Erroneous primitive reflexes produce abnormal and asymmetrical muscle tone leading to subluxation complexes and dysfunctional motion. Learn for yourself how these primitive reflexes work and find out how to address them quickly to optimize your patient's human performance.

Receptor Based Solutions™ describes functionally useful physiological reflexes that are easy to check on every patient at every office visit. These examinations are very important because according to the medical literature, the presence of these reflexes suggests potential brain damage from stroke or traumatic injury, and their presence is considered abnormal when present beyond the age they are expected to be integrated. However, it is not the presence of these reflexes that is clinically important; rather it is their atypical display that indicates the potential for brain damage. The atypical presence of one or more of these reflexes together with the absence of the higher level reactions in older children or adults can have a significant impact on muscle tone, the ability to isolate movements, balance, and functional skills such as feeding and ambulation. Here is the issue: Each of these reflexes should be present in their expected array. But since much of this erroneous display is secondary to abnormal sensory input, treating the deafferentation properly often resolves the abnormal display.

Receptor Based Solutions™ will help the doctor integrate the primitive reflex patterns into a functional understanding of posture and its various displays. The merger of these reflexes amongst themselves produces seven uniquely individual displays—one of which is the neutral and proper upright posture—that the doctor will learn to progressively test and rebuild.

When these reflexes perform according to their original design they will display themselves as intended, and when they fail it will be obvious. A failed reflex response has a very high probability of indicating that other problems are inherent in the more rostral neuraxis; i.e., the cerebellum, basal ganglia, thalamus, and cerebral cortex, and each has its associated autonomic concomitants. *Receptor Based Solutions*™ will both help you address these fundamental reflex issues and your patients reshape their humanity.

Receptor Based Solutions™ will give the doctor greater understanding about this innate framework for movement and depict ways to help that movement become appropriately functional. Each one of your patients can reach their highest level of human expression because you have read and applied *Receptor Based Solutions*™.

The Receptor-Dependent Nervous System

The Input that Creates a Response

Introduction

The chiropractic philosophy of 1895 was consistent with the prevailing scientific ideas. It explained the art and science to the level of neurological understanding that existed at that time. Chiropractic's founder, D.D. Palmer's first descriptions of chiropractic were much like that of osteopathy, established a decade earlier. Both philosophies considered the body as a "machine" whose parts could be manipulated to produce a drugless cure. These were the same days when Wilhelm Roentgen, a German professor of physics had just discovered electromagnetic radiation in the range known as X-rays and the "reticular theory" was still the popular thought in neurology.

The reticular theory, which was suggested by a German anatomist Joseph von Gerlach in 1871, and popularized by the Nobel laureate Italian physician Camillo Golgi, held that the whole nervous system— including the brain—was made up of a singly entwined network. The idea, however, was disproved by the subsequent observations of the Spanish pathologist Ramón y Cajal, which were summed up as "the neuron doctrine." Using the very same techniques that Golgi used, Cajal confirmed that discrete neurons did exist, thereby strengthening the concept of the growing neuron doctrine. The neuron theory turned out to be the correct description of the nervous system while the reticular theory was rejected. Subsequently, Golgi and Cajal were jointly awarded the Nobel Prize in Physiology or Medicine in 1906, "*in recognition of their work on the structure of the nervous system.*"

In the 1950s the electron microscope finally confirmed the existence of individual neurons in the central nervous system, and the existence of gaps in between neurons called the "synapse." With that, the reticular theory was finally put to rest.

Although the chiropractic philosophy was adequate for the time, it was relatively simplistic and inadequate when compared to our current level of understanding. Today, chiropractic can be very appropriately explained in the light of sensory receptor physiology rather than the archaic ideas of nerve pressure. Sensory receptor function is at the core of human neurology. Understanding the function of receptors is vital to our understanding of chiropractic. Unlike most new ideas in literature, basic receptor physiology is relatively simple to understand.

Explaining Sensory Input

Because patient education is so important in our practices, I would like to explain what I say to help my patient's understand about how their nervous system works and why muscle function is so important to brain stimulation. The explanation is very simple and it maintains accuracy.

First, spend just a moment and look at the flow chart below. Consider how each item flows into the next one. Its continuity displays a fundamental physiological concept that few doctors apply in their practices, but once the doctor understands this flow the whole picture becomes second nature.

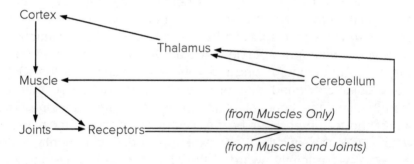

Figure 3: Muscle-brain interactions involve joints and their receptors

This is what I say as I build the Muscle-Brain Interaction diagram (Figure 3):

Figure 4: Muscles move joints

"*It is important to understand that when muscles contract, bones and joints move. Muscles move joints; joints do not move muscles.* [And I write the word "Muscle" (Figure 4), and then I draw an arrow down and write the word "Joints" underneath it.]

In many ways, a joint acts like a hinge. Anytime a muscle contracts, it moves two bones closer together. To move the bones further apart, a second muscle (the one that pulls against the first one; the antagonist) must contract while the first muscle relaxes so the bones can move the other way. The muscles that move the joints must work reciprocally.

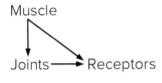

Figure 5: Muscles and joints stimulate receptors

As the joint moves, the muscles and joints (pointing to each word as I speak) *send signals to the brain by way of sensory receptors* [then I write "Receptors" (Figure 5) and draw arrows to it from "Muscle" and "Joints"] that monitor the movement and position of the joints.

These receptors send their signals through both subconscious and conscious pathways. The subconscious receptor signals first arrive at an area of the brain called the cerebellum (also known as the "little brain"; Figure 6), located just above the base of your skull inside your head. The cerebellum is an error comparer. It constantly blends the subconscious signals it receives with those sent from other muscles from various parts of the body. This allows the brain to coordinate body movements.

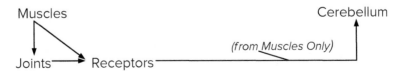

Figure 6: The cerebellum receives receptor input from muscle

The cerebellum sends its unconscious motor signals to two places. One set of cerebellar signals goes to the muscles (Figure 7) on the same side of the body to provide modulation. (The cerebellum plays an important role in motor control, contributing to coordination, precision, and accurate timing. It may also be involved in some cognitive functions such as attention and language, and in regulating fear and pleasure responses, but its movement-related functions are the most solidly established.)

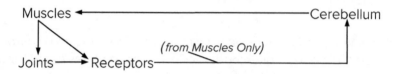

Figure 7: The cerebellum unconsciously controls muscles

Other receptors, like the balance mechanisms in the ears, are part of the vestibular system and also exchange messages with the cerebellum. When working properly, this whole mechanism allows your muscles to keep you standing up straight and move you around with efficiency without even having to think about it.

Two other areas that subconsciously control muscle functions are the hearing mechanisms in the ears, and vision. For example, if someone walks up beside you and speaks, you will reflexively turn and look toward them. It is the ability of these systems to work together subconsciously that allows the muscles to function properly.

The function of the thalamus (known as "the inner chamber," located between the cerebral cortex and midbrain; Figure 8) is almost totally based upon the stimulation of sensory receptors. The cerebellum sends its unconscious input to the thalamus...

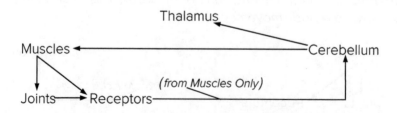

Figure 8: The cerebellum unconsciously stimulates the thalamus

...as well, the thalamus receives conscious receptor signals from the muscles and joints (Figure 9). The thalamus acts as a "switchboard," relaying sensory and motor signals to and from the cerebral cortex. It also influences the regulation of consciousness, sleep, and alertness. All sensory information must pass through the thalamus before it reaches the brain, except for the sense of smell, which goes somewhere else.

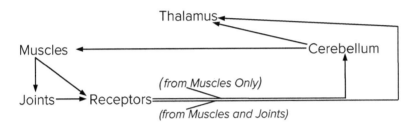

*Figure 9: Muscle and joint receptors stimulate
the thalamus, as does the cerebellum*

This all happens in the blink of an eye. The thalamus integrates the conscious messages with the subconscious input from the cerebellum...

...and the thalamus forwards its input to cortex (Figure 10).

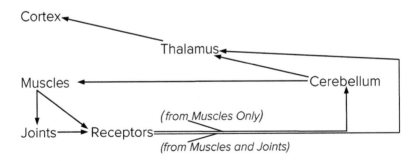

Figure 10: The thalamus forwards its input to the cortex

The cortex is the principal area that controls the muscle response based on all the sensory input it receives..."

...so that the brain can both consciously and unconsciously control the muscles to move the joints (Figure 11).

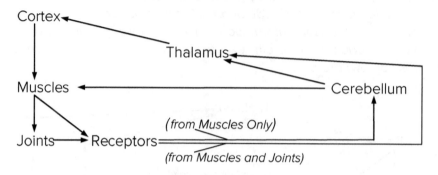

Figure 11: The cortical control of muscles

Take a Look Backwards

At this point, I ask the patient if they have any questions on this chart so far. If there are, I will explain it again. If not, I will review the chart backwards.

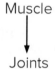

Figure 12: Joint input from the muscles

"As you can see, this whole mechanism must be balanced. The joints are solely dependent upon the muscles for their stability (Figure 12).
(At this point it often becomes clear to the patient that the muscles have to work properly so the joints move according to their preprogrammed plan. If the muscles contract inappropriately, the joints will be imbalanced, and both of these erroneous inputs compromise the signals that reach the thalamus and brain.)

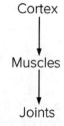

Figure 13: Muscles are controlled by the cortex

The muscles are dependent upon the ability of the cerebrum (the cortex; Figure 13) to work at its highest level of function, because it is the cortex's responsibility to control all the areas underneath it; the cortex's main function is inhibitory, i.e., it is designed to control or modify the rest of the body.

40

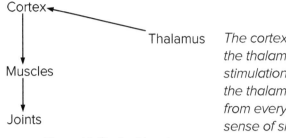

The cortex is dependent on the thalamus' overall level of stimulation (Figure 14), and the thalamus receives input from everywhere except the sense of smell.

Figure 14: Cortical input from the thalamus

Further, the thalamus is dependent upon two areas for its stimulation. The first such input is from the unconscious signals that proceed from the cerebellum (Figure 15), which must be at their optimal level of stimulation...

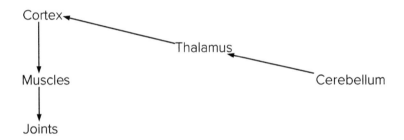

Figure 15: The thalamus receives input from thecerebellum

...because the muscles depend upon cerebellar input to maintain structural stability (Figure 16).

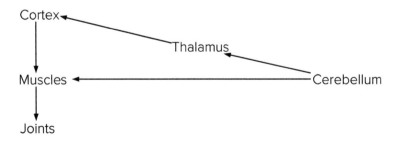

Figure 16: Unconsciousmuscle input from the cerebellum

The second input to the thalamus comes from the receptor stimulation that arises from the more conscious receptors found in the muscles and joints that are responsible for joint stability (Figure 17).

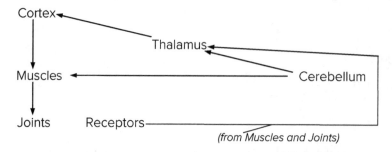

Figure 17: Thalamic input from the muscle and joint receptors

Finally, the cerebellum receives afferents from the muscle receptors of the same side (Figure 18).

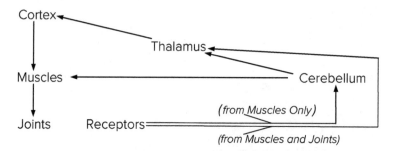

Figure 18: The cerebellum receives input from the muscle receptors

Both of these receptors are stimulated by muscles and joints, being responsible for a high degree of reciprocal joint position sense (Figure 19).

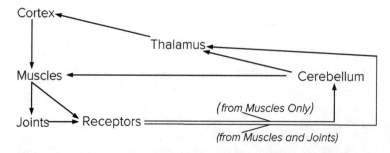

Figure 19: Receptor input from both the muscles and joints

Lastly, I expand the chart forward again, this time with a twist of dysfunction.

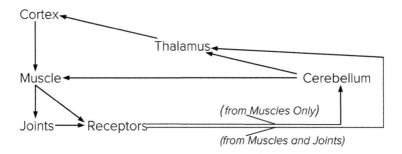

Figure 20: The schematic of muscle and joint receptor stimulation to the cerebellum, thalamus and cortex to both consciously and subconsciously control muscles

"If the subconscious and conscious receptor signals to the cerebellum and thalamus (Figure 20) are inadequate because the joint's movement is flawed, (i.e., the joints have lost their reciprocity— the trait of use and counterbalance) then the information sent to the cortex will also be flawed making its role fall short of its optimum. Moreover, cortical compromise causes inaccurate motor signals to reach the muscles, which leads to a loss of joint integrity and a further breakdown in the quality of sensory signals to the brain. It is a degenerative cycle that impacts whole body function. We call this deafferentation, a reduction in the sensory input to an area that should have otherwise been stimulated.

This breakdown causes an imbalanced body to send mistimed signals. The nervous system is sensitive to its internal timing because the human nervous system is designed to contain organization and flow. The human nervous system was meant for order and precision, not disorder and breakdown. Mistimed sensory input begets mistimed outflow. In other words, the brain can only respond to what it receives. When the brain receives flawed incoming signals it responds with defective outgoing signals to wherever these signals would go, including to the glands and organs, and that sets up hormone and other functional imbalances.

In order to correct this physiological breakdown, the doctor must understand how to address the muscles and joints to encourage the right kind of receptor stimulation to the brain that resets the optimal muscle function.

Review the Chart Again

"The key to interrupting this vicious cycle breakdown is to physically interact with the muscles and joints in a way that works with the patient's functional individuality. This interaction has the highest probability of stimulating the greatest number of joint receptors possible, instantly exciting the cerebellum and thalamus, and they stimulate the cortex. Increasing cortical function helps it regain its inhibitory control over the muscles and joints. This leads to more normal receptor stimulation to the cerebellum, thalamus and brain, and back again to the muscles, stabilizing the brain's functions. This increases joint position sense and steadiness, and reestablishes the brain's control over the body".

It is my hope and goal that every patient would understand this cycle of structure and function so that they can know why it is important for their health that they reclaim their optimal human performance. The more people know about how their body works the more excited they will be about rejuvenating their health, and they will in turn tell others of their potential renewal.

The Hormonal Connection; *Preserving the Bridge*

Muscle function and joint motion set the foundation for hormone control. Optimal afferentation is the stimulus that keeps the human nervous system healthy and strong. Vibrant, cognitive and physical health depends upon a healthy nervous system.

Remember that we learned that the higher cortical centers inhibit those centers underneath them. Now we will learn that the bridge between the structural and endocrine (hormonal) systems lies in the connection between the thalamus and hypothalamus. This is where the joint signals of muscle performance are changed into various neurochemical *releasing hormones* (RH; also known as releasing factors) that each control the release of a specific hormone. The more integrity there is between the thalamus and hypothalamus, the healthier will be the bridge between the nerves and hormones.

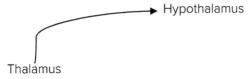

Thalamus

Figure 21: Thalamic and hypothalamic interconnection

Simply stated, the thalamus oversees the hypothalamus (Figure 21). While there are many associated circumstances, the thalamus is designed to have a controlling influence on the way the hypothalamus works. To say it differently, the hypothalamus is outranked by the thalamus. The hypothalamus performs relative to the commands given it by the thalamus.

The Hypothalamus

Let's take a brief look at the hypothalamus (the "under room", or "under chamber"). It is an extremely important, yet almond sized collection of distinct nuclei with other less anatomically distinct areas that sits in the brain's centerline just below the thalamus, and just above the brainstem. One of the most important functions of the hypothalamus is to link the nervous system to the endocrine system via the pituitary gland (hypophysis) and each individual hypothalamic nuclei has its own specific purpose with a variety of responsibilities.

The hypothalamus is responsible for certain metabolic processes and other activities of the autonomic nervous system. It manages the overall functions of the nervous system that are not under voluntary control, making it is the highest level of the entire nervous system that helps activate, control and integrate the endocrine, autonomic, and behavioral functions. In short, the hypothalamus is known as the master gland.

The hypothalamus synthesizes and secretes certain neurohormones, often called releasing hormones or hypothalamic hormones, which in turn stimulate or inhibit the secretion of pituitary hormones involved in:

- The control of daily cycles that influence the physiological state and behavior
- Autonomic control
- Temperature regulation
- Thirst and control of body water
- Appetite control

- Sexual behavior and reproduction
- Endocrine control
- Sleep and wakefulness
- Stress response
- Emotional reactions

...including fertility.

Releasing Hormones

The human endocrine system is a closed system. It was designed to only handle a certain amount of each hormone and no more. When the feedback systems inform the hypothalamus that there is enough of a particular (or a combination of specific) hormone, the hypothalamus cuts back its production of releasing hormones to ample amounts that maintain that system's specific needs. If a person ingests hormones—i.e., like the ones prescribed by most medical infertility specialists—the endocrine system will respond by cutting back its own hormone production in order to maintain what it considers to meet the systemic needs, but the imbalance of one hormone often means the disparity of another related hormone.

Here is an overview of how the endocrine system is designed to work: The hypothalamus secretes releasing hormones (RHs) that are destined for the anterior pituitary, which is right underneath it (Figure 22). The main RHs secreted by the hypothalamus are:

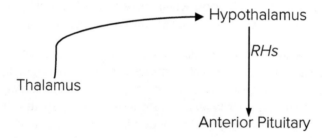

Figure 22: The hypothalamus stimulates the anterior pituitary

- Gonadotropin-releasing hormone (GnRH), also known as Luteinizing-hormone-releasing hormone (LHRH) and luliberin,
- Thyrotropin-releasing hormone (TRH), also known as thyroliberin or protirelin,
- Corticotropin-releasing hormone (CRH), also known as corticoliberin,
- Growth hormone-releasing hormone (GHRH), also known as somatoliberin or somatocrinin.

Now follow along here because this is very important (Figure 23): The thalamus (1) stimulates the hypothalamus (2), which secretes RHs that biochemically stimulate the anterior pituitary (3) causing it to secrete *a stimulating hormone* (SH) specific for each target gland (4).

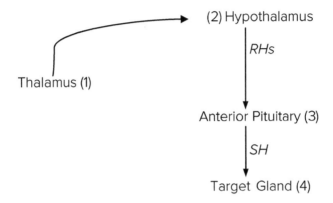

Figure 23: The anterior pituitary stimulates the target gland

(Figure 24) That target gland (4) responds by sending its specific hormone—or hormones—back to the hypothalamus (2), which is the target gland's (4) way of informing the hypothalamus (2) that it did as it was instructed to do...

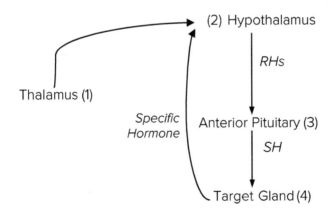

Figure 24: The target gland gives feedback to the hypothalamus

...and the hypothalamus (2) responds (Figure 25) by slowing its release of the RHs (5), and therefore SHs, which eventually brings the whole system to a functional balance.

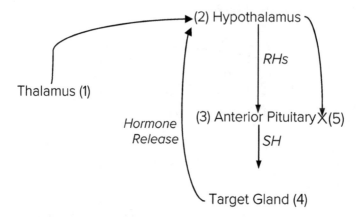

Figure 25: The hypothalamus reduces its output of releasing hormones

Review this process again because this hormonal system is fearfully and wonderfully created, and extremely sensitive.

Hormone Similarities

Let's take a look at the hormone system again, but this time we will review it backwards.

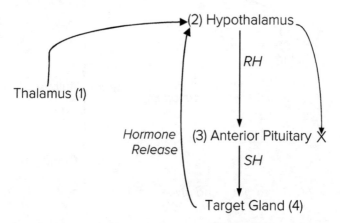

Figure 26: An overview of the hormonal feedback loop

All hormones (Figure 26) are ultimately released from a target organ (4), which received a SH from the anterior pituitary (3), which is stimulated by a RH that the anterior pituitary received from the hypothalamus (2) that is under the hierarchical control of the thalamus (1), which (when connected to the previous diagram, Figure 27) is stimulated via incoming conscious and unconscious neurological signals from the cerebellum and other receptors that arise in muscle, ultimately in response to joint and muscle stimulation.

Putting the Two Flow Charts Together

When these two flow charts (Figure 20, between the muscles, cerebellum, thalamus, cortex and back again to the muscles, and Figure 26, which details the flow from the thalamus to the hypothalamus, pituitary, and the target glands) are linked together, it looks like this:

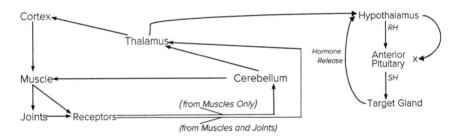

Figure 27: A schematic of the muscle and joint receptor influence over hormonal balance

The Outflow from the Brain

Up until this point we have focused on the receptor signals from the joints and muscles to the cerebellum, thalamus, and brain, and from the thalamus to the hypothalamus, which turns its nerve signals into releasing hormones that manage the pituitary. These hierarchical controls are inherent in the human system where each center above modulates the systems below it to the end that the lower centers remain under the controls of the segments that are higher up the tiered chain. As we described, the cortex exerts its modulatory control over the thalamus, and the thalamus has modulatory controls over the hypothalamus.

Now, this point is very important to our whole discussion: Of the entire outflow that comes from the brain, only 10% of that outflow goes back to the muscles. Ninety percent of all the signals that come from the brain go to the organs. That means that the outflowing information from the brain has a greater influence on the organs than it does to the muscles, and if the doctor only pays attention to the muscles, he or she will miss the brain's most valuable expression—the autonomic concomitants.

Consistent with the other regimented controls, the mesencephalon— which is a portion of the central nervous system that remains undifferentiated throughout life (Table 17)—has an inhibitory influence over an area below it called the reticular centers of the upper part of the brainstem (Figure 2), just inside the base of the skull. Finally, these lower brainstem centers have their own inhibitory influence over spinal cord centers, particularly of the anterior horn, that allow and disallow certain motor responses. Any disruption of these inhibitory cascades sets up dysfunction that should have otherwise been inhibited. These interferences display themselves in the muscles that move the joints, whose receptor signals feed back to the cerebellum and thalamus as we have previously discussed.

Summary

This discussion gives an overview of muscles and the receptors then to the brain, and the thalamus has upon both hormones and descending nerve signals that go to the muscles, and ultimately back to the brain.

Where, before, we discussed the pituitary underneath the hypothalamus, there is another descending cascade of hypothalamic control that involves nerves, which neurologically inhibits the mesencephalon (Figure 2). This is the area where vision makes its first post-retinal synaptic connection. The mesencephalon contains a special area (the Edinger-Wesphal nucleus) that is the highest representation of all autonomic function, which influences the brainstem and various areas of the spinal cord.

Deafferentation, "Pinched Nerves" and the Chiropractic Adjustment

Introduction

For just over 100 years, chiropractic promoted the concept of "anatomic displacements" that gave rise to inflammation, and thereby, to dis-ease. These displacements eventually came to be known as "subluxations" that were not only something of diagnostic value, but they were also the major foundation of the profession. When Palmer made his first observations in 1895, the subluxation theory was in step with the science of the day but his theories were a quantum leap forward.

Then, in 1934, when Cajal—the purported father of modern neuroscience—was awarded the Nobel Prize for his work on the neuron theory—which conceptualized that the nervous system was made up of discrete individual cells—it was clear that the subluxation with its resultant "pinched nerves" was not an explanation for the overwhelming benefits that chiropractic provides. Simply put, when the nervous system was thought of as being reticular (i.e., without interruption), a case could be made for the pinched nerve theory. As it became understood that neurons are in synaptic contact, the pinched nerve theory was no longer a viable model. However, the pinched nerve theory's demise did not distract from chiropractic's successes as a viable healthcare option. And again, the chiropractic profession found itself beyond the abilities of the day's scientific explanation.

Based on the disproof of the pinched nerve theory, critics felt that they had grounds to criticize chiropractic's scientific grounds. They screamed "placebo," "spontaneous remission," and "quackery." Consequently, and in their attempt to explain the effectiveness of chiropractic care, supporters often fell back to the science of 1895 and the philosophy upon which chiropractic was founded, but it had already been "disproved" by Cajal's discoveries. The only thing that was clear was that neither side could adequately explain what happened to the nervous system when a patient received an adjustment.

Chiropractic's Coming of Age

For the past several decades, the chiropractic profession has built clinical success upon clinical success, but there was as yet no viable model to explain the mechanism of those successes. While in other healing arts the lack of a scientific model had not necessarily been considered a problem (e.g., aspirin was in use for 70 years before its mechanism was fully explained), rather it merely showed the necessity for research. As far as chiropractic's critics were concerned, the lack of a viable model was proof that there was no scientific explanation. The simple fact is that neither chiropractic physicians, nor anyone else in the health care community was able to explain the far-reaching effects of chiropractic adjustments until the explosion in neurologic knowledge that has occurred since the early 1980s.

Now, as a result of irrefutable and multidisciplinary research, all reasonable scientific literature indicates that the entire human nervous system is receptor-based. That is, the sensory (afferent) nerves from joint mechanoreceptors are the foundation for maintaining the nervous system's ability to function as an integrated unit. It is organized in a rostral-caudal fashion. That is, the greatest preponderance of joint mechanoreceptors is in the spine, with the highest population of those receptors in the upper spine with a decreasing presence as we reach the lower spine. Further, the upper extremity has a higher neurologic priority than the lower extremity; likewise, there is a higher population of joint mechanoreceptors in the upper part of the upper extremity relative to the lower part of the upper extremity.

Pinched Nerves

Actually, nerves seldom become pinched, but if one were pinched it would quickly (usually begins within 24–36 hours of a lesion) undergo Wallerian degeneration, retrograde chromatolysis,

52

ultimately resulting in the death of its axons, and subsequently the neurons themselves. The death of a nerve cell happens quickly; in nanoseconds. Those neurons whose degeneration proceeds to cell death do not recover their function, and that function remains lost to the patient, whereas functional deafferentation can be reversed through increasing the afferents of joint mechanoreceptors.

Here is a case in point: A medical doctor shared the story of a patient who came to him complaining of lower back pain of several months duration with resulting sciatica that involved his left leg all the way to his ankle. The doctor suspected that his patient had a lumbar disc problem so he ordered an MRI and he said the findings confirmed his diagnosis.

The doctor further related that he explained the issues to this patient and prescribed some medication to help his patient with his pain. The doctor went on to say that the patient listened to the explanation and understood how to take the medication. When the doctor finished, the patient looked down at the medication and back at the doctor and asked, "Which one of these medications will un-pinch the nerve?"

The doctor said that he described that one medication was a muscle relaxer and the other was an anti-inflammatory drug. Understanding what he had just heard, the patient again asked the doctor, "Which one will un-pinch the pinching in my nerve?" At that, the doctor said that he just stood there for a moment struck by the logic of his patient's question and confessed he did not have the answer.

The doctor said, "I told him that the muscle relaxer was designed to release the tension in his lower back muscles to let the joints move better and that the anti-inflammatory drug might reduce the swelling in the tissues around the nerve and that that might help ease the pain, too. Despite how profound that answer sounded," the doctor continued, "I began to question its reality."

The upshot of the story is that the pinched nerve diagnosis is rendered to patients every day. If the muscle relaxers and pain killers do not do the trick, the next step is a steroid. Steroids are considered standard procedure for the medical community and in many areas wavering from these steps could be considered grounds for medical malpractice, because this is just what medical doctors do to treat a pinched nerve.

Muscle relaxers are designed to relax muscles and pain killers are designed to kill pain. In most cases these medications are not the answer because one tight muscle only indicates that another muscle related to that same joint is not pulling like it should to balance the joint. Further, if a patient has pain it probably means that the signals that would otherwise forbid the realization of the pain are not as strong as they could be, and, as we shall see, they too relate to dysfunctional joints.

Deafferentation

When a vertebra is stuck within its normal range of motion and is unable to move through that normal range of motion (the definition of a subluxation), a quantum of joint mechanoreceptor afferents are lost (deafferentation), and the functional continuity of the neuraxis suffers. The disturbance created by that deafferentation can be detected not only at the local spinal cord level [affecting several different aspects of cord function (Table 1), including the intermediolateral cell column and/or anterior horn, just to name a few areas, and causing reflexogenic myospasms and autonomic concomitants], but also more rostrally.

A deafferentation reduces the central integration of the neuraxis at a variety of levels including but not limited to the receptor,

Table 1: Twelve Cord-Centered Primary Afferent Events:

For every afferent signal that reaches the cord, 12 things happen simultaneously.

All primary afferents:

- **Are excitatory to the intermediolateral cell column.** This allows for dilation of arterioles to muscles, capillaries to skin, piloerector tissue and sweat glands
- Inhibit pain (excites inhibitory interneurons to inhibit nociception)
- Excite alpha motor neurons of the homologous muscles, i.e., right upper extremity flexors
- Inhibit alpha motor neurons of antagonistic muscles, i.e., right upper extremity extensors
- Excite left upper extremity extensors
- Inhibit left upper extremity flexors
- Excite right lower extremity extensors
- Inhibit right lower extremity flexors
- Excite left lower extremity flexors
- Inhibit left lower extremity extensors
- Ascend to the brainstem
- Ascend to the cerebellum

spinal cord, cerebellum, basal ganglia, thalamus and/or cortex, any or all of which can disturb the functional capacities of the deafferentated structure. Thus, it is not "un-pinching a nerve" that results in the affects we see following a chiropractic adjustment. Rather, the stimulation of the joint mechanoreceptors with a fast stretch coupled manipulation increases the primary afferentation from these joints, returning neural physiology to a more normalized central state of integration.

Pain can be defined as the cognitive realization of inappropriate joint motion. Now stay with me here: Pain is the conscious awareness of *nociception* (the unconscious process that deciphers, stores and makes meaning out of harmful, poisonous, or very unpleasant stimuli that have the potential to damage tissue), which is always present; everyone has nociception. Stated another way joint motion knocks out pain. More appropriately, *reciprocal* joint motion is what inhibits nociception in the dorsal aspect of the spinal cord.

A Place to Hide

The largest fibers inside a nerve carry *proprioception* (the unconscious realization of the neighboring parts of one's body in space) while the smallest fibers convey nociception. Therefore, a pinched nerve is probably not the cause pain, because if a nerve were to be pinched the smallest fibers would essentially find hiding places amongst the larger diameter fibers. Any effect of "pinching" a nerve fundamentally displays itself in a proprioceptive breakdown that, as a result of that nerve's inability to bring the spinal cord interneurons to threshold, allows the passage of nociceptive input that eventually reaches conscious perception, which the patient describes as pain. Moreover, if a nerve were truly pinched there would be an accompanying disuse or denervation type atrophy of the muscles fibers related to that nerve.

Besides, the benefits one receives as a result of an appropriately delivered chiropractic adjustment are not because of the biomechanical movement of a joint that un-pinches a nerve. Rather, a properly coupled manipulation depolarizes joint mechanoreceptors to re-afferentate the associated spinal nerves and their concomitant internuncial pools that presynaptically inhibit the passage of nociceptive afferents. Further, these primary afferents also stimulate the more rostral neuraxis that results in the positive and almost instantaneous physiologic changes seen daily in chiropractic practice.

Effects of the Coupled Manipulation

When we consider the most common pain control remedies, the effect of coupled depolarization of joint mechanoreceptors results in an afferent input to the apical interneurons of the dorsal horn that is far more efficient than drugs or other types of medication. While drugs bathe the whole nervous system in their effects, joint manipulation is very specific in its neurological influence.

These neurons that are stimulated by joint mechanoreceptor manipulation send their axons to axoaxonally hyperpolarize the primary neurons of the nociceptive (e.g., a noxious stimulus; a type of neural process that encodes and processes noxious stimuli; the sense that allows people to experience pain via stimuli that have the potential to damage tissue) system, driving them away from threshold (or toward potassium equilibrium potential), resulting in a hyperpolarization that reduces the nociceptive bombardment of second order neurons at the basal spinal nucleus. This inversely downgrades the quantum of pain experienced by the patient relative to the number of mechanoreceptors depolarized (i.e., the greater numbers of mechanoreceptors depolarized, the less the pain experienced by the patient. This inhibitory effect requires reciprocity). Further, mechanoreceptor stimulation simultaneously brings about the depolarization of signals from the thalamus to the hypothalamus, to the reticular formation, and onto the apical internuncial pool in the cord that will drive the *central integrative state* (CIS; originally described by Carrick) to postsynaptically inhibit nociceptive concomitants in the anterior horn through the interneuronal synapses.

The concept that the human nervous system has a central integrative state (CIS) is unique to the philosophy of chiropractic. It was developed by Frederick Carrick, DC, PhD, Professor of Clinical Neurology and the founder of the Carrick Institute for Graduate Studies; some consider him the father of functional neurology.

Carrick's concepts have opened a vast arena for discussing the possibilities of functional factors that may influence the internal condition of a nerve and even the effect of those influences upon the whole picture of nervous system performance as it relates to the consequences of treatment for the human condition.

Since all joint mechanoreceptor afferentation must pass through the thalamus before it reaches the cortex, primary perceptual experience is dependent upon thalamic integrity, which is itself dependent upon the integrity of the mechanoreceptors. Thus, a decrease in joint mechanoreceptor activity will cause a shift in the central state of both the thalamic and cortical integration and consequently a resultant shift toward potassium equilibrium potential, bringing about a concomitant decrease in cortical activity. Therefore, increasing joint mechanoreceptor activity increases kinesthetic joint position sense, postural relationships, the ability to think, remember, see, hear, etc. Indeed, coupled joint mechanoreceptor stimulation has a profound effect on the patient's ability to express their unique humanism.

Volitional motor activity is also dependent upon cortical integrity, which is dependent upon thalamic depolarization to the cortex, which is largely a result of the mechanoreceptor afferent system. Even though the descending modulation through the globus pallidus, caudate, putamen and mesencephalic motor centers is beyond the scope of this book, suffice it to say that there are feedback loops from the cortex to the basal ganglia and back to the thalamus before they are reintroduced to the cortex again in order to compare that information to the existing CIS of the thalamus. It is by increasing mechanoreceptor afferentation that it is possible to increase thalamic integrity, thereby increasing feedback to the centerline neuraxial centers that increase the central state of mesencephalic integration.

It is also essential to consider other mechanoreceptor collaterals that fire disynaptically to the cerebellum, upon which postural integrity is largely dependent through their stimulation of the vestibular system. Its rostral concomitants affect mesencephalic motor centers compensating for decreases in cortical volitional activity, and increasing bombardment of the alpha motoneurons and interneurons of the spinal cord at every level.

The autonomic nervous system is depolarized as a consequence of that extrapyramidal bombardment through the midbrain and brainstem, from the thalamus and hypothalamus to the reticular formation and that continues through the spinal cord, as well as concomitant second order neuronal bombardment in reflexogenic pathways in the cord.

Summary

The present day science and art of chiropractic is well realized through multidisciplinary research literature, which strongly substantiates the foundations of chiropractic. We now know that the coupled manual manipulation of any joint—especially zygapophyseal joints of the spine—evokes a very large population of mechanoreceptor afferents. Stimulating these areas in a coupled fashion produces remarkable effects throughout the entire neuraxis. Chiropractic patients can immediately experience their magnificence. The reduction of pain and the enhanced primary perceptual experiences, motor performance, autonomic function, certainly the patient's ability to more appropriately express their unique humanism are all majestically affected by the functional state of the joint mechanoreceptors.

Since it is biomechanical integrity that gives us the highest populations of mechanoreceptor afferents, any forfeiture of that preprogrammed performance via aberrant biomechanical relationships will result in a deafferentation of that mechanoreceptor input with resulting quantitative pathology or malfunction in the patient's ability to alleviate pain, appreciate primary perceptual experience, modulate joint reciprocity, and the ability to move and control vital functions. Therefore, it is evident that our very humanism is dependent upon the integrity of joint mechanoreceptor afferentation, which is best preserved by the well-trained Functional Neurologist.

An Overview of the Clinical Aspects of Vertebral Coupling

Introduction

The clinical aspects of vertebral coupling are important in order to understand the concept of functional afferentation of the neuraxis and the clinical manifestations of deafferentation. This chapter deals with the neurological implications of both coupling and dyscoupling from a physiological and a neurological perspective.

A nine view cervical series made up of a standard five views with a right and left oblique, and a right and left lateral bending taken at 72 inches.

Similarly, a seven view lumbar series contains a standard five view lumbar series with right and left lateral bending views.

Radiology

Plain radiographs are generally used to diagnose and/or evaluate the extent of major or overt osseous disorders such as congenital anomalies, canal stenosis, fractures, dislocations or erosive bone pathologies and arthritis. However, they can also be used to examine a solitary segment of the full range of spinal motion.

When radiologically examining the cervical and lumbar spines from a functional perspective, it is clinically prudent to perform a nine view cervical and/or seven view lumber series. In the cervical spine, this should consist of the standard five view cervical series with the addition of right and left obliques, and right and left lateral bending views. The lumbar series should contain the five standard views as well as right and left lateral bending views. The rational for these procedures will follow.

Cartesian Nomenclature

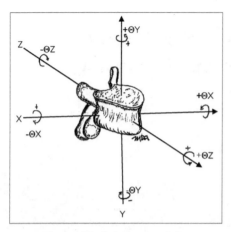

Figure 28: Schematic of the Cartesian System as applied to a vertebral position, designating its instantaneous axes of rotation (IAR).

Any individual vertebra or a group of vertebrae can move through three cardinal ranges of motion designated by the Greek symbol theta ("θ"), which means, "rotation" (Figure 28). This system is named after its originator, Rene Descartes, and is called the "Cartesian" system. It represents a universally recognized coordinate system of nomenclature. It uses three intersecting coordinate planes along the "X", "Y" and "Z" axes to specify a directional position each relative to the others.

The Cartesian system is represented by two horizontal planes and one vertical plane, all of which run perpendicular to each other. The X and Z axes both run horizontally. The X-axis goes from left to right, while the Z-axis goes from posterior to anterior. The vertical, or Y-axis, goes from inferior to superior (Figure 28).

This same coordinate system can be used to designate the body's position in space as well as in describing body movement. Physiologically, if movement takes place *around* the X-axis in a positive ("+") direction, it is considered to be a flexion-type movement. Conversely, movement around the X-axis in a negative ("-") direction would be extension. Therefore, when viewed from the right, flexion of the cervical spine is termed +θX axial rotation. The movement of the cervical spine around a -θX axial rotation is considered to be extension.

The same idea applies to movement *around* the Z-axis. When viewed from behind, a +θZ axial rotation is considered to be a right lateral bend, whereas a -θZ axial rotation is a left lateral bend—or a clockwise and counter-clockwise range of motion of the vertebra, respectively; this same idea could also apply to a group of vertebrae.

If movement takes place *around* the Y-axis in a positive ("+") direction— as viewed from the feet—it is a clockwise movement, and is designated

+θY axial torque. A −θY axial torque is a counter-clockwise movement around the Y-axis.

Translatory movements are seen along the same axes, but not preceded by the Greek symbol "θ." They are simply in a positive ("+") or negative ("-") direction, along the path of its designation.

A +X translation is movement from left to right, and a -X translation is movement from right to left. Following the same mode of thinking, a +Z translation is motion from posterior to anterior, and a -Z translation is movement from anterior to posterior. Finally, a +Y translation is a movement from caudal to rostral, white a -Y translation is a movement from rostral to caudal.

Application of these principles can be tricky at first, but with repeated use it becomes second nature. Cartesian nomenclature is very specific relative to other non-standard methods of designating vertebral position, the direction and/or the limitation of that movement. While there are various nomenclatures used within chiropractic to designate vertebral and total body movement, this Cartesian system does not require the understanding of any specific technique in order to realize the position of vertebral subluxation. Likewise, the position of subluxation and the direction of manipulation can be readily understood by anyone in the medical field even if they are unfamiliar with adjustive techniques.

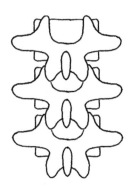

Figure 29: Normal zygapophyseal alignment of the lumbar spine

Vertebral Coupling

The human neuraxis is designed to receive information from its internal and external environments and respond to it. The primary uptake of this information, in this case concerning the internal environment is from the periphery (so called because it is outside the *central* nervous system) through the joint mechanoreceptors—proprioceptors—which are generated as a result of musculoskeletal maneuvers. These afferents are carried via electrical signals through a succession of neurons to the central-most parts of the nervous system. Consequently, the motor response is transmitted back to the muscles and organs, completing a means for biomechanical feedback.

Fundamental to this process of receiving and transmitting information are the zygapophyseal joint mechanoreceptors (Figure 29) whose graded, nonpropagated stimulation should ideally summate both spatially and temporally in order to reach threshold. Once threshold is met, their associated axons propagate a nongraded afferent signal along their large diameter (type Ia) axons in order to bring the rostral neuraxis to its functional state.

Despite the apparent logic of this fundamental process, the fact that this process can be interrupted is often overlooked. These primary afferents can be modified—either for better or for worse—at various functional levels, especially in the receptor, spinal cord, cerebellum, basal ganglia, thalamus, cortex, or distally at the end organ, or at any other area the signal may become deafferentated.

The term "coupling" refers to the normal and physiologic action of a vertebra or group of vertebrae around or along any or a combination of the three cardinal axes of movement (Figure 30). Another term for the same movement is the "Instantaneous Axis of Rotation" (or "IAR"). It has to do with the movement of each individual vertebra, as well as one vertebra relative to its immediate neighbors.

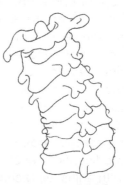

Figure 30: Coupled cervical motion

Cervical Coupling

Normally, for example, when laterally bending the cervical spine to the right, the spinous processes must couple toward the convexity of the curve. When laterally bending the cervical spine to the left, the whole mechanism reverses. The rule: Cervical vertebrae should properly couple to the side opposite of the lateral bend, or toward the convexity of the curve.

Coupled motion produces compression of the facets on the concavity of the movement and expansion of the facets on the convexity of the movement, causing different types of excitation of the zygapophyseal

The most fundamental spinal movement is flexion/extension. The next most essential movement is lateral bending. The most complicated spinal motion is torque. If flexion/extension and lateral bending are stable, then torque is most likely harmless. However, if torque takes place on a spine whose flexion/extension and/or lateral bending movements are unstable, then the torqueing motion will most likely cause joint pathology.

joint mechanoreceptors on each side and driving them toward sodium equilibrium potential, or excitation. This causes the afferentation of the higher centers whose tissues lie at the termination of each afferent segment of its neurologic tract, including the arousal of postsynaptic potentials with a concomitant facilitation of muscle function commensurate with that motion, and the resultant afferentation of higher neurologic centers.

Lumbar Coupling

Because of the prioritized rostral-to-caudal orientation of the neuraxis, the process of cervical spinal coupling has a much higher priority than that of the lumbar spine, but the latter cannot be discounted. The former movement sets precedence for the latter, and the latter must be able to function homologously with the former.

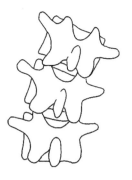

Figure 31: Coupled lumbar movement

For example, when the lumbar spine laterally bends to the right, the spinous processes must couple toward the concavity of the curve—to the right (Figure 31). Likewise, when the lumbar spine laterally bends to the left the spinous processes must couple toward the concavity of the curve—to the left. Lumbar coupling is opposite from that coupling seen in the cervical spine. The rule: Lumbar vertebrae properly couple toward the side of the lateral bend, or toward the concavity of the curve. Lumbar dyscoupling (Figure 32) can sensitize the free nerve endings in the area to several chemicals that cause noxious stimulation to free nerve endings and subsequent pain.

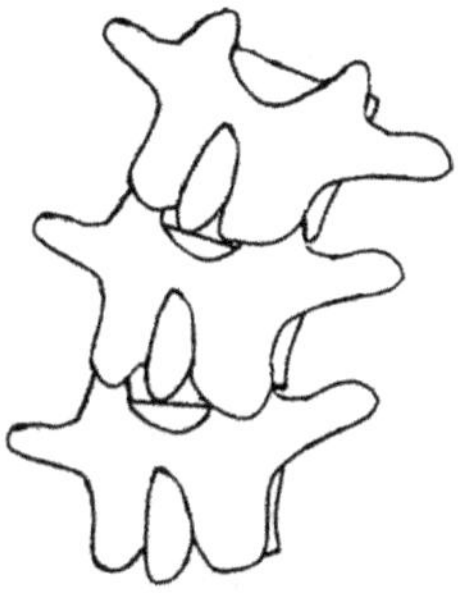

Figure 32: Dyscoupled lumbar motion

Purposeful Movement

Purposeful joint movement requires the coordinated action of many paraspinal muscles. Their primary afferents reach the rostral neuraxis to affect the motor outflow that facilitates coupled motion. Even the relatively simple volitional act of lateral bending the head on the neck requires a reciprocity that coordinates the facilitation and inhibition of dozens of independent yet homologous muscles so they can act in concert and manage a single movement. This entire mechanism is believed to be managed chiefly by the cerebellum.

> Deafferentation contributes to the inability of joint mechanoreceptors to presynaptically inhibit nociceptive reflexogenic afferents leading to the very real probability of the realization of pain.

However, if the vertebral segments demonstrate a dyscoupled motion (taking into account only joint motion), it causes those facets on the concavity of the curve to respond as if they were undergoing expansion and those on the convexity of the curve to respond as if they were undergoing compression. Although the joint mechanoreceptors still function as they were designed, they are not brought to threshold efficiently. This causes a relative decrease in the number of excitatory postsynaptic potentials and a concomitant inability to summate the sensory afferents either spatially or temporally. Therefore, there is a relative increase in inhibitory postsynaptic potentials that lead to compromised function and the hyperpolarization of higher centers. In effect, the dyscoupling displays to the higher centers that the muscles on the concavity of the curve are relaxing while those on the convexity of the curve are contracting. This results in a dysfunctional afferentation of the higher centers, driving them toward potassium equilibrium potential (inhibition) with the production of an aberrant population of postsynaptic potentials and the resultant hyperpolarization of those postsynaptic tissues. This mechanism is clinically known as "deafferentation."

Deafferentation

Deafferentation is the result of compromised joint motion, which leads to biomechanical deficits and the breakdown of polyanionic glycosaminoglycans of joint cartilage. These chemicals depolarize the nociceptive type III and IV afferent fibers that are found in the intertransverse ligaments, the collateral ligaments of the appendicular skeleton and lattice-like plexuses or free nerve endings of various articular tissues respectively. This produces nociceptive reflexogenic myospasms and the very real probability of concomitant painful experiences. At the same time, there is a compensatory paucity of the modulatory effect of the higher centers on the alpha motoneurons in the anterior horn cells of the spinal cord. As well, the dysfunctional modulatory mechanisms lead to autonomic concomitants through the inhibition of the disynaptic postsynaptic inhibitory pathways through the intermediolateral cell column.

No matter its location, dyscoupling indicates the high probability of reflexogenic myospasm, and the resultant deafferentation of the neuraxis. Myospasms generate uncoupled signals to the supraspinal centers, causing the muscles to function contrary to their intended purpose, leading to further deafferentation that arises as a result of these myospasms. The normal vertebral movement is restricted and the spinous processes remain fixed in their position, prohibiting coupled motion. Clinically, dyscoupled movement mimics movement to the uncoupled side, causing a relative expansion of the facets on the concavity of the curve with a concomitant relative compression of the facets on the convexity of the curve. It is as if the spine neurologically laterally bent to the one side when it physically laterally bent to the other. A completely dysfunctional movement!

The brain responds to dyscoupled movement by causing the muscles to perform a motion that is consistent with the deafferentation. Because of the pathological movement the motor response is unnatural to that which should physiologically occur. That is, the muscles that should be contracting on the concavity of the lateral bend become relaxed, and those on the convexity of the curve contract when they should be relaxed. This failure of musculoskeletal reciprocity leads to the destruction of joint cartilage with the potential for further joint deafferentation and the probable realization of pain, which is the result of the noxious stimulation of free nerve endings that ultimately reach conscious levels and all the neurological responses consistent with that stimulation.

The Chemical Stimulation of Free Nerve Endings

Several chemicals cause noxious stimulation to free nerve endings. Among them are histamine, polyanionic glycosaminoglycans, lactic acid, bradykinins, prostaglandin E, and 5-hydroxytryptamine. No matter the source, if these chemicals find their way to nervous tissue, the result is nociception. Its conscious and unconscious ramifications and resultant myospasms are due to an inhibition of postsynaptic inhibition in the dorsal horn and/or inhibition of disynaptic postsynaptic inhibition from the interneuron from the intermediolateral cell column.

Abnormal Instantaneous Axes of Rotation

The quality of movement of each vertebral segment can be defined by evaluating the instantaneous axes of rotation (IAR) of each spinal segment in question. Generally, symptomatic patients can be characterized as having a wider than normal distribution of their IAR's. The suggestion is that patients with spinal pain exhibit abnormal patterns of vertebral movement that could be detected by determining their IAR's both in the cervical and lumbar regions.

A substantial proportion of patients with spinal pain do exhibit abnormal IAR, but not necessarily does it relate to the area of perceived pain. This occurs in the context of patients in whom plain radiography was otherwise normal. A large proportion, although not all patients with spinal pain, exhibit abnormal IARs of spinal joints in areas remote to that of their pain. This abnormality does not reveal the source of the patient's pain, but it does correlate with the presence of pain. Pain is a completely personal and emotional experience and cannot be considered directly proportional to the amount of tissue destruction. Therefore, pain should more correctly be thought of as a consequence of deafferentation rather than tissue damage.

Foremost, this relationship of IARs to the experience of pain indicates that an abnormal IAR constitutes an objective marker for the presence of pain. An abnormal IAR indicates a biomechanical disturbance that occasionally occurs in people who experience no pain, but it is significantly more frequently in patients who do experience pain. Nociceptive myospasm has the capacity to reduce the vertebral range of motion and to alter the IAR; this is in fact a common denominator.

However, the abnormal IAR is not the only cause of deafferentation. It signals the inability to inhibit nociception and/or pain because of a decreased afferent signal from the large diameter axons, which arise from joint mechanoreceptors. Nociceptive reflexogenic myospasms can also result from biomechanical deficits resulting in a biochemical failure.

Palpation of Coupling

Palpation of cervical and/or lumbar coupling is relatively easy. Have the patient lie supine. The $+\theta Y$ axial rotation of C7, for example, can be examined by pressing the right transverse process from posterior to anterior. This causes a $+Z$ translation of that transverse process and *mimics* a $-Z$ axial rotation of C7 and the entire cervical spine, because that is the way the cervical spine moves with a $+\theta Z$ axial rotation with a simultaneous $-\theta Y$ axial torque. At the same time, press the spinous process of C7 from left to right in order to *mimic* $+\theta Y$ axial torque. This is the way the vertebra should move if it is coupling properly. Any limitation of this motion in any direction represents the high probability that the range of motion of that vertebra is limited through $-\theta Z$ axial rotation and $+\theta Y$ axial torque, and that the functional movement of that level is dyscoupled.

The procedure for the lumbar vertebra is similar. However, if the range of motion is limited through $+\theta Z$ axial rotation, it will also be limited through $+\theta Y$ axial torque by virtue of the mechanism of its coupling. *Remember,* the lumbar vertebrae couple in a direction opposite those of the cervical spine.

Treatment

A dysfunctional IAR with concomitant nociception indicates the need for osseous manipulation in order to increase excitatory postsynaptic potentials and decrease inhibitory postsynaptic potentials both spatially and temporally to those areas of the neuraxis requiring a greater level of function. This is done via fast stretch coupled manual chiropractic reductive techniques *directed toward those joints that demonstrate* a *resistance to motion.*

The fast stretch coupled reduction causes the inhibition of the nociceptive myospasms via the excitation of type Ib afferents from Golgi tendon organs. There is a simultaneous stimulation of type I and type II joint mechanoreceptors found in zygapophyseal joints of the axial skeleton. The result is in an increased probability of a spatially and temporally summated barrage of afferentation to the spinal cord, cerebellum, thalamus and cerebrum. There is also a concomitant presynaptic inhibition of nociceptive reflexogenic afferents in the dorsal horn of the spinal cord (Figure 33). Further, through disynaptic postsynaptic pathways, the same large diameter axon's synaptic connection to the intermediolateral cell column normalizes autonomic concomitants. This reestablishes the modulation of corticospinal and corticobulbar pathways via the alpha motoneurons of the ventral horn.

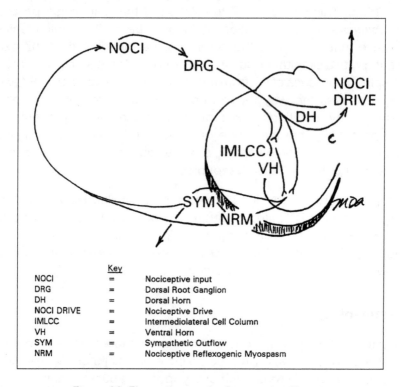

Figure 33: The pathway of reflexogenic afferents

The treatment may also require the application of physical therapy, the use of oxygen, dietary changes, and other parts of a balanced treatment program. However, the intent of this paper is to deal with the structural ramifications of vertebral coupling. Therefore, other treatment programs will not be addressed at this time, but they should not be overlooked when indicated.

Summary

The functional human vertebral column moves in a highly predictable manner. It does so because of the functional barrage of the axial muscles and joint mechanoreceptors as well as via the afferentation of those other more rostral centers that make us human. It enables balance and stability, and the ability to inhibit nociception and/or pain. On the other hand, if deafferentation arises as a result of dyscoupled movement for example, degenerative changes and pain should be expected.

Dyscoupling and/or an abnormal IAR constitute objective markers for the presence of pain. They indicate a biomechanical disturbance that occurs in those people who are apparently pain free, but it appears to be significantly more frequent in patients with pain of many kinds. Muscle spasm has the capacity to reduce the functional range of motion and to alter the IAR, resulting in further deafferentation and resultant reflexogenic myospasm. The cycle is vicious! This is common in all pain syndromes, and in the vast majority of cases can be corrected with *coupled* chiropractic manipulative techniques consistent with the normal IAR of the involved osseous structures with the intent to introduce the highest probability of afferentation of the neuraxis globally.

True health is the ability to maintain a functional nature in the face of adversity. There are many ways to confront these adversities. The most beneficial way to affect the functional status of the human neuraxis even to its most rostral centers is via the application of *coupled* spinal motion and the normalization of afferent signals to the most rostral centers of the neuraxis.

Section II

Receptor Based Solutions™ for Your Patients

Receptor Based Solutions™ for Your Balance

The Highest Incidence of Accidental
Death is from Incidental Falls

Introduction

It would be nice if the sensory input from one side of the body would be equal to the input from the same part on the other side of the body. Imagine what it would be like if the input from the eyes, ears, and muscles were all symmetrical. The anatomical illustrations of the eyes and their associated muscles always look pleasantly symmetrical in the books as do those of the semicircular canals and skeletal muscles. The structures on each side seem to perfectly reflect each other. All things being equal, when the input from one side of the body matches the input from the other side of

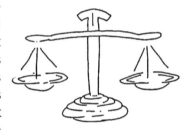

Figure 34: Balance and counterbalance

the body, the brain senses balance and it responds similarly (Figure 34). Equilateral feedback would be a tremendous contribution to a balanced brain. But in reality, none of these feedback systems are as equally proportioned as the pictures and their explanations found in anatomy books.

The certainty of asymmetrical input sets up the potential for, more appropriately the probability of, brain hemisphericity that displays itself in sensory and motor dysfunction. That sensory and motor imbalance is called a *mismatch*, and mismatch happens.

Balance Systems

We humans use three systems for balance: Our eyes for visual input, our inner ears for vestibular input—both the right and left side systems are encased within the bones of the skull, which moves relative to the trunk—and our cerebellum for joint position sense either at rest or in motion, otherwise known as proprioception. These three systems must work in unison for us to make sense of our environment.

It is ultimately important to remember that muscles move joints, not the other way around. In general, muscles respond to gravity and perform relative to joint motion.

The cerebellar system is housed in the skull but is not contained within bone as are the semicircular canals of the inner ear. The cerebellar primary afferents arise in the muscles and are the sole source of sensory input to the cerebellum and the majority of that muscle input is axial relative to gravity. The neck muscle proprioceptors—afferents from joint mechanoreceptors—which give some of the highest priority input to the brain, stabilize the head relative to gaze, upright posture, and the position of the trunk. Orientation and stabilization of the trunk axis—the largest axis—is critical during leg movements and during locomotion, especially when the supporting structure oscillates.

It would be nice if these three inputs from the eyes, ears, and muscles were all symmetrical, but, in reality, they are not. Actually, the structure of each of these systems varies from the pictures in anatomy books. Books make these systems look so good, but that is not how it is in real life. Because of their placements, input from one part of your body regularly differs from that input that arises from the same part on the opposite side of the body, and these variances must be resolved.

The eye muscles cannot move the same way on each side like other muscles can. In each position of gaze, a muscle of one eye is "yoked" with a muscle of the other eye to move the eyes, together, in a certain direction. The ear's semicircular mechanisms never match from side to side because turning the head one way causes one type of semicircular stimulation and the opposite type on the other side. The sum of the two movements must cancel each other out in order to maintain balance. Any discrepancy—or mismatch—from one eye or ear to the other, or amongst themselves, sets up pathological input that must be handled by the individual's nervous system—the cerebellum, basal ganglia, and cerebral cortex. (The truth is that mismatched sensory input is more the rule than the exception.) Most of the time the nervous system is able to handle slight differences, but there is a limit to their ability to adapt. The more sensory dysfunction we have, the more complicated balance becomes.

Upright Posture

People often ask me how they developed their functional problems; how did they create their pathologies? The answer is that these problems began as a consequence of imbalanced sensory input relative to gravity. Recall the 12 things that happen every time a primary afferent reaches the cord (Table 1). These events are predictable. The breakdown of this display is the cause of every mistimed neurological response.

The patient's posture most often becomes unstable when they develop neurological timing errors. When the signals from one of these three areas do not match those signals from the other two areas—or from one side of the body to the other side—the nervous system must recalibrate the error; that is a cerebellar process. For that split second any deviation from balance can cause a person to be at risk of falling from a mismatch related to the vestibular system.

Our antigravity muscles are mainly of the extensor type, their tone being significant to their ability to perceive their stimulation. The antigravity muscles are designed to resist gravity's push and keep us upright; they oppose the probability of a fall. Antigravity muscles serve as an interface with the external world for perception and action. The sensory input from these three particular systems provides orientation relative to space as a frame of reference.

If the muscles on one side of our body have more tone than those same muscles on the other side of our body, the posture adapts in various ways, and we develop a structural and/or functional perturbation, i.e., a postural antalgia. Imbalanced muscle tone causes postural and resultant cortical sensory errors with a higher probability that gravity can topple us at any significant distraction. In the presence of a sensory mismatch, any stumble or bump that creates further muscle imbalance can lead to a devastating functional breakdown. At that moment, we may not be able to step quickly or turn fast enough to stop a serious fall.

Balance and Proprioception

Balance is organized globally—it involves the entire structure—mainly for equilibrium control. It is maintained as the postural boundaries are managed inside the base of support. During movement, the center of support is basically maintained at the ankle joint by the muscles that control the feet. This whole interaction centers in the pelvis, allowing dynamic posture changes relative to the constantly changing demands of gravity; the lower body makes steady postural changes underneath the faster moving upper body.

Balance is also organized in a segmental fashion, for example, to orient the head and neck relative to space. This gives a reference for sensitivity and realization. In reality, there is one kinematic chain from feet to head but it is not controlled by a single functional unit. Its maintenance requires the input from several individual segments—particularly from the eyes, ears, and centerline—each tied to the next one by a set of muscles that has its own central and peripheral controls aimed at maintaining its reference to the segment.

In general, the nerves that sense joint motion (the various types of proprioceptive afferents) are never silent. There is always some joint signal going somewhere and doing something. The systems that are designed to work together exchange their information while those systems that are meant to counterbalance that work exchange their information, all the signals from the joints and muscles working together so the brain unconsciously knows where the body is in space at any given moment.

Balanced afferentation and an appropriate motor response is always the goal. However, imbalanced sensory input always results in an asymmetrical motor response that pulls the joint toward the tighter muscles. It is not unusual for the motor signals that go to muscles on one side of the body to tend to have a greater influence than the motor signals that go to the muscles on the other side of the body. These structural imbalances set up vicious cycles of mismatched sensory input to the brain and motor outflow to the muscles. In they come and out they go; sensory and motor chains stimulate each other with wonderful succession.

Recall that we previously stated that the eyes and ears are housed inside the head and the muscles of the neck generate the highest priority signal to the brain. The way the head sits on the neck, for example, plays a deep-seated role in the interpretation of all sensory input. Therefore, because of this three pronged input and our individualized response to them, no two people who have the same symptoms can ever receive the same treatment.

The head's position depends upon the signals that come from the eyes, ears, and spinal muscles; the neck moves the head, and trunk follows suit. Balance has to do with managing feedback. To be in balance, posture and movement have to work together. Imbalance happens when sensory and motor mismatches make the brain think something is happening other than what really is happening. From both balance and imbalance, the way the muscles work is the result of sensation.

> The human brain considers its response relative to total body function rather than relative to an individual muscle's performance.

Balance Has Limits

Did you ever try to stand with both feet on the ground and lean as far as you can in any direction without falling? Can you lean further one way than another? Balance is the unconscious sensation you generate that keeps you from submitting to gravity.

It may seem elementary, but it is nonetheless important to point out, that one of the essentials to upright posture is the ability to stay within your own personal protective limits of balance. Pushing those barriers can lead to risky instabilities.

A person is either aware of their body position in space or they are not, there is no middle ground. Balance comes about when the brain is able to interpret all the sensory input in a way that is appropriate relative to reality. But what happens when the brain interprets the sensory input relative to what it thinks is reality, but that reality does not exist? Those with a sensory pathology may think they know where they are in space, but their sensation has a high probability of mismatch relative to certainty. Erroneous input will set up a sensory conflict that tends to generate a motor response inconsistent with their body is in space, increasing the probability of falling and an increased potential for injury.

This tendency to fall is most prevalent in the young; it declines in the teens, and then increases again from the mid-twenties. By age 60, statistics show that one in three people will take a fall. In reality, these sensory inconsistencies can be diagnosed and treated, reducing the potential for falling and injury.

Do not let your patients become a statistic. They are probably totally unaware of their potential to fall until it is too late. Physically examine each patient right away and know where they stand. Ask their family and friends about their balance, too, and perhaps you—the doctor—can prevent an injury and better yet, save a life.

Summary

Balance is an unconscious event perceived through the eyes, ears, and paraspinal muscles, and interpreted by the cerebellum, basal ganglia, and cerebral cortex. It depends upon a balanced input and motor response, and subject to how the head sits on the neck. Any confusing sensory signal upsets the whole process and leads to erroneous subconscious posturing and an increased tendency to fall.

The fact that one person's balance issues are different than another person's demands that each be treated relative to their unique needs. Treating all people with balance issues the same way could only lead to further mismatches. Anyone with balance issues should seek out the doctor who can best address each patient's individual needs and stick with them.

Case Study #1

History and Presenting Complaints: John (66y) complained of right lower back pain after trimming his trees for three days and that his energy was lower than he liked. He also said the vision in his right eye had been slowly deteriorating the past 10-12 years.

Exam Findings: John has been in overall good health for several years. He walks seven miles twice daily within his personal aerobic rate, but one important thing stood out during his physical exam. Stroking the sole of his foot with a sharp object functionally inhibited the proximal rectus femoris ipsilaterally, and the sartorius appeared to be functionally inhibited bilaterally.

The MMTs showed a normal display when John covered his left eye, but all the original muscle findings remained when he covered his right eye, indicating that his brain was able to interpret the input from his right eye better than it did from the left eye.

Next, while his right eye was covered, John counted backward from 100 by 7's, but the dysfunction persisted. With his right eye still covered, he hummed a new tune aloud. This second test made all the MMTs display as anticipated.

Clinical Impression: It appeared that the image from John's left eye was unconsciously troubling him (a possible strabismus) and that was supposedly his better eye. That dysfunction appeared to cause a dysfunctional sensory input and muscle display. Introducing a right brain activity appeared to enhance the stimulation to that side of his brain, producing a more appropriate motor response, indicating that the sensory and motor systems matched and the MMTs performed according to their original design.

Treatment Plan: We used some special red/blue hemifield goggles to stimulate and hold John's right cortex on display while patching his right eye. Then we looked for structural findings that would increase the functional abilities of his right brain.

Response to Care: After the treatment, we removed the goggles and patch. The muscles were retested and the patient displayed appropriate findings—his fMMTs all had their anticipated display.

Discussion: Through certain functional neurological pathways, John's right lower back was quite possibly the result of a deafferentated right brain secondary to a structural dysfunction on the left side. This is called a soft pyramidal display or a stroke antalgia.

Consider the bounds of stability provided by balance. John's presentation was as if his nervous system sensed that he had swayed too far forward and left relative to his environment, and his muscles in his lower back tightened to keeping him from tending too far forward. The sensory mismatch teased him into subconsciously thinking that he needed to be pulled back and to the right, when, in fact, he was physically in no danger of falling forward.

Receptor Based Solutions™ for Your Deep Tendon Reflexes

Functional Display of the Myotatic Stretch Reflex

Introduction

The CNS regulates both internal and external environments—the autonomic and somatosensory components, respectively—each have their own sensory and motor divisions. Of all the somatosensory reflexes, the spinal reflexes are the simplest, and are classified into superficial, visceral, and deep reflexes. While both the superficial reflexes and visceral reflexes are clinically important, this article will deal with the deep tendon reflexes (DTRs).

The deep tendon (more commonly called the myotatic stretch) reflexes are rapid excitatory responses of a muscle following stretch. It is typically performed during a standard neurology exam. A DTR can also be performed using fMMT techniques. The stretch response should not only demonstrate the characteristic muscle contraction relative to the stretch of its tendon, but it should also be accompanied by a concomitant crossed cord reaction and by autonomic concomitants, such

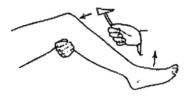

Figure 35: The patellar reflex

as an appropriate blood supply. For example, it is essential for a muscle to receive its requisite blood supply when it contracts and when it relaxes. Blood nourishes every muscle to keep them viable. However, a muscle's function and its associated autonomic responses may not always be synchronized. These autonomic concomitants are sometimes mismatched with their associated muscle's demand and the nourishment is slow to be delivered. This can result in joint instability and muscle pain.

The Stretch Reflex

The stretch reflex is fundamental to the involuntary control of posture and movement. The first observations of stretch reflexes were reported as early as 1751, by Robert Whytt. Experiments since then have revealed that the stretch reflex is a complex muscle reaction with various timing issues occurring at different intervals following a muscle stretch. As a result, there remains controversy regarding the stretch reflex's functional role. Even after more than 260 years there is still not clear understanding about what is happening. However, there appears to be agreement that the stretch reflexes can be modified in a task appropriate manner.

The Patellar Reflex

The patellar reflex (Figure 35) is a clinical and classic example of the monosynaptic reflex arc (Figure 36). Striking the patellar tendon—the insertion of the quadriceps—with a reflex hammer causes an almost instant extensor display in its related muscle. The knee jerk is the result of an arc that goes from the insertion tendon of the rectus femoris being tapped to the spinal cord, then monosynaptically back to the muscle.

Theoretically, a monosynaptic reflex has no interneuron in the pathway leading to facilitation of the stimulated muscle. However, in reality there is an inhibitory interneuron used to simultaneously inhibit the antagonistic hamstring muscle, which allows for the extension of the leg on the thigh; the characteristic "kick".

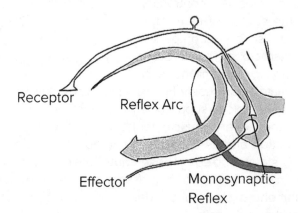

Figure 36: A monosynaptic reflex arc

This patellar or "knee jerk" DTR appears to be a kind of stretch reflex the presence and integrity of which is a common part of even the most basic neurological exam; it is an important sign of neurological development and function. It assesses the functional integrity of the central and peripheral reflex pathways. It is commonly considered that a very strong DTR response (hyperreflexia) is typically indicative of an upper motor neuron lesion while a hypoactive response (hyporeflexia) to stimulation may typically be indicative of a lower motor neuron lesion.

Specifically, the peripheral receptors (i.e., the muscle spindles) perceive and grade the stimulus. Once that stimulus meets the receptor's threshold, the neuron transmits an afferent impulse fully and completely in the sensory fibers of the femoral nerve leading to its first integration in the lumbar spinal cord and brain stem. One aspect of the sensory neuron makes a single connection onto a motor neuron in the ventral horn of the spinal cord that conducts an efferent response to the rectus femoris muscle, for example, triggering its contraction and the characteristic knee jerk.

The repeated activation of a synapse increases its efficiency or plasticity. The DTRs can also be upgraded as during repetitive activities like practicing a movement, or when linked with autonomic responses related to conditioning. Both the DTR and its autonomic concomitants have to do with cerebellar consequences. And they can be functionally altered by the same mechanisms. This upgrading helps improve awareness throughout the reaction's homologous columns. Further, any reaction inconsistent with the homologous consequences can also be evaluated by fMMTs.

Fundamentals: Tapping the patellar tendon should cause the foot to kick one time and then the reflex should be extinguished. Coupled with the kick is a concomitant increased blood supply to the muscle because it is performing work. This demonstrates a coordinated segmental response between the DTR and the autonomic nervous system, i.e., the autonomic concomitants.

Associated Conditions: The pathological absence or decrease of the patellar reflex is known as Westphal's sign (the clinical correlate of the absence or decrease of patellar reflex or knee jerk). It is a characteristic finding in tabes dorsalis, a type of neuro-syphilis.

The reflex's absence has other clinical significance used in determining neurological disorders or diseases such as receptor damage, peripheral nerve disease involving the dorsal (sensory) columns of the spinal cord and cerebellar lesions, lesions present within the motor cortex of the brain or the pyramidal tracts that is combined with muscular spasms, or complete interruption of sensory and/or motor impulse transmission in the femoral nerve.

Extension Strategy

Patients often present with a hyperreflexia of the lower limb(s). There may also be a hyperreflexia in the upper limb and the combinations of display will most probably involve homologous columns.

Examining the functional condition of the knee may involve a functional facilitation where a functional inhibition would be expected. This represents an increased extensor tone and indicates that the extremity in question has assumed an extension strategy inconsistent with the anticipated reciprocal display making activities like transfers and ambulation very difficult.

Postural Strategy

When a patient presents with a hyporeflexia of the lower limb, especially at the knee, it is associated with a concomitant flexion postural strategy of the ipsilateral hip and ankle. This lower extremity posture represents a tactical response to gravity that may be either functional or adaptive. It may inhibit the patient's ability to bear weight with a potential for fall-type injury should a perturbation occur that propels the patient in a manner inconsistent with their acquired posture.

Summary

Seat your patient on your table and test the patellar reflexes. Note your findings. Now lay that patient supine and functionally examine the rectus femoris muscle with a straight leg. Again, note your findings. Now, with that patient's legs relaxed tap the patellar tendon again and retest that muscle. Did that muscle's function change? Both the functional facilitation of a previously functionally inhibited rectus femoris muscle and the functional inhibition of a previously functionally facilitated rectus femoris muscle indicate the need for some sort of intervention. The point is that you just demonstrated a functional DTR response. Just like the deep tendon stimulation of the patellar reflex in the seated position displays a motor response, specific muscle stimulation—in this case a supine DTR of the same patellar tendon—in any posture suggests the condition of the neuraxis.

The following erroneous DTR case study is important because it suggests that there was some functional misperception in Matthew's nervous system that could have been anywhere along the reflex arc from the tendon of reception to the anterior horn of the cord and back to the muscle. It is one key to further understanding the condition of the patient's nervous system and should encourage the doctor to look further for the cause.

Case Study #2

History and Presenting Complaints: Matthew (20y) presented in my office complaining of right knee pain of gradual onset. There appeared to be no known trauma or other etiology.

Exam Findings: Among other tests, we examined the muscles of Matthew's knees with both standard neurological reflex tests and fMMT. Both the patellar reflexes and basic MMTs responded as anticipated. However, more advanced fMMTs of the rectus femoris showed that tapping the insertion of the left patellar tendon caused a normal functional facilitation of that rectus femoris while tapping the insertion of the right patellar tendon caused a functional inhibition of that muscle. Typically, each MMT would have caused functional facilitation of the ipsilateral rectus femoris.

Clinical Impression: The absence of knee jerk is not unusual in the clinical setting with no indications of other hard pathological signs. However, now that we understand more about this clinical presentation, its absence does make one wonder about the integrity of the reflex arc. Relative to the exam findings, we could say that Matthew's quadriceps DTR display was abnormal. Consider that the CIS of the reflex has changed from neutral where the facilitory and inhibitory stimuli are balanced, to one of conditional inhibition..In essence, we might consider that the segmental functions of the anterior horn have been driven away from that which is considered normal and the muscle displays a functional inhibition.

Treatment Plan: In this case, the clinical indications were to adjust Matthew's right foot.

Response to Care: Adjusting the patient's right foot resulted in the immediate functional facilitation of his right rectus femoris.

Discussion: The patellar tendon reflex has been thought to help maintain upright posture. The reflex tests the function of the femoral nerve and spinal cord segments L2-L4.

Striking the patellar tendon on either side appeared to cause an ipsilateral knee jerk response of equal grade. Further, testing the left rectus femoris immediately after tapping its patellar tendon appeared to show a nominal response; the rectus femoris displayed a functional facilitation. However, testing the right rectus femoris immediately after tapping its patellar tendon appeared to indicate that the test either did not meet or it exceeded that tendon's functional capacity; the muscle appeared to be functionally inhibited. As a result, we could say that the right rectus femoris was unable to meet the demands of fMMT.

In theory, the left femoral nerve reflex arc appeared to summate in the receptor and update quickly in the spinal cord because the purposeful timing of these links appeared to be functioning properly. However, that of the right reflex arc did not appear to summate properly. It neither responded with the anticipated knee jerk reaction, nor did the rectus femoris muscle appear to update properly indicating that the afferent signal expired somewhere between the receptor, the spinal cord, and the effector in the associated muscle. Another possibility is that the connections from the more rostral neuraxis that control the anterior horn of the spinal cord inhibited the reflex (i.e., the CIS of the final common pathway was driven toward functional inhibition, a potassium equilibrium potential).

While there are many possible explanations for this dysfunction, the essence comes down to timing. Just because the reflex arc is drawn toward or away from stability does not mean that it will work like that every time. There must be some allowance for functional interference and some process to find and correct that interference.

Receptor Based Solutions™ for Your Tonic Neck Reflex

Taking up the "Fencing Posture"

Introduction

It is quite commonplace that most everything written about primitive reflexes indicates that they eventually disappear as a child moves through their normal development. Their normal displays are important signs of a typical and maturing nervous system when present at their expected milestones. Some writings imply that the "unexpected return" of a primitive reflex is significant, but these views deserve reconsideration. Actually, the absence—or the inappropriate display—of an expected primitive reflex at any given stage is thought to imply some abnormal neurological function. As we shall see, the primitive reflexes should never unexpectedly return; the truth is they should never go away if the nervous system is intact.

Look up the tonic neck reflexes (TNR) on the internet and you will find videos of doctors turning the heads of healthy babies from side to side to watch how their postures change. Turning their head one way facilitates some muscles while inhibiting others and turning their head the other way makes the opposite happen. It is fascinating.

The Tonic Neck Reflexes

Primitive reflexes like the TNRs are inborn actions originating in the CNS. While they are correctly exhibited by neurotypical infants—and contrary to many of the common academic perspectives—this author believes the TNR, as well as many of the other primitive reflexes, to also be demonstrably intact in functionally competent adults in response to particular stimuli.

Moreover, it seems more appropriate that rather than "disappearing", these primitive reflexes are gradually incorporated into the normal human neurological fabric by the maturation of the frontal lobes. Similarly, any frontal lobe demise will eventually allow "escape" of the normal cortical modulatory controls, which enables the display of cortical release signs (CRSs).

If, like many authors believe, the TNR were to actually disappear by a child's first birthday the human fabric would be missing an essential component to upright posture and functional stability.

Two Tonic Neck Reflexes

The primitive neck reflexes are actually of two types: The Asymmetrical (Figure 37) and the Symmetrical (Figures 38 and 39) Tonic Neck Reflexes (ATNR and STNR, respectively) (Table 2).

The neck reflexes arise via stimulation of joint receptors in the neck (especially around the atlantooccipital and atlantoaxial joints) when the head is inclined forward, backward, or sideward, or rotated to either side. That is, for example with the ATNR, turning the head to the right should cause functional facilitation of the extensors on the side toward head rotation and the functional facilitation of the flexors on the side opposite head rotation. Conversely, the ATNR response causes a functional inhibition of both the flexors on the side toward head rotation and of the extensors on the side opposite head rotation. This rule applies to both upper and lower extremities (Figure 37).

In the absence of TNR influence, the postural demands of bipedal carriage would be impossible. While a person can certainly move around despite ATNR dysfunction, their operative display would be "something other than human".

The Asymmetrical Tonic Neck Reflex

The first of the two TNRs to appear is the ATNR. The ATNR is commonly displayed in newborn humans, but it is also found in other mammals.

It has been shown that turning the head of an infant younger than six months of age to one side will display an archer's posture. Similarly, turning the infant's head to the other side causes the opposite display. While this posture is appropriate, many different authors say that the ATNR normally vanishes by the child's first birthday, but that observation is functionally and demonstrably inconsistent with reality in clinical practice. A neurotypical child may no longer automatically display an ATNR, but the muscle response to head rotation can be demonstrated at any age. In fact, the ATNR can be demonstrated to persist throughout life and it is a fundamental part of neurological integrity and a tool for neurological examination.

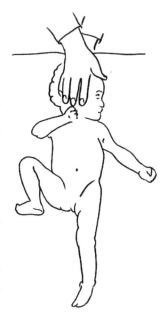

Figure 37: The Asymmetrical Tonic Neck Reflex

The ATNR is fundamental to and inseparably fused with core stability and balance; the right and left ATNR reinforce each other in their effects on the upper extremities and oppose each other in their effects on the lower extremities. However, the aspects of steadiness seem to be the more dominant response for lower extremity patterning.

The ATNRs help modulate postural tone, orienting the leg and trunk posture as a function either of the neck or pelvis position in space. Relative to the ATNR rule, we will see in the upcoming case study that the patient's original psoas display was other than that which would be expected as humanly normal, or "other than human" and therefore pathological. The patient's ATNR dysfunction indicated that a very important low back stabilizer was working contrary to its original programming, and that has a very high probability of indicating a concomitant functional upper cervical and/or occipital problem.

A dysfunctional ATNR displays as a functional compromise of any normal display. For example, when the patient turns their head to the right, there should be functional facilitation of the extensors on the side of head rotation and a functional inhibition of the flexors on that same side. Any display that reveals an *f*MMT other than what is anticipated should always be considered to be dysfunctional.

Further examination of this dysfunctional ATNR display clinically indicated that the patient's low back stability was the result of inappropriate cervical receptor stimulation—i.e., uncoupled cervical spinal motion. Additionally, it suggested that upper body performance may have been a more primary problem than lower body movement; the lower body tends to follow the upper body.

Moreover, the ATNR is not an isolated part of the human neurological design. The ATNR cannot function independently from the rest of the nervous system. Subsequent to cervical joint mechanoreceptor stimulation, afferent signals continue from the cervical cord to rise to the cerebellum, midbrain, basal ganglia, and cerebral cortex. Faulty sensory input from these cord segments means an inability to presynaptically inhibit nociceptive reflexogenic afferents and subsequent related motor errors, compromised autonomic concomitants, structural problems, and the probable conscious perception of pain.

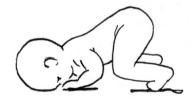

Figure 38: Symmetrical Tonic Neck Reflex with head in flexion.

Upon flexion of the head on the neck there is a simultaneous flexion of the fore limbs and hands and extension of the hind limbs.

The Symmetrical Tonic Neck Reflex

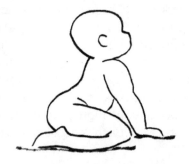

Figure 39: Symmetrical Tonic Neck Reflex with head in extension.

When the head extends upon the neck there is a simultaneous extension of the fore limbs and flexion of the hind limbs, bilaterally with plantar flexion of the foot.

The STNR provides for the separation of body movements between the upper and lower halves of the body, which develops subsequent to the STNR; it is a cycle.

The STNR is considered to be the normal progression of infants from a more immature neurological state to their early locomotion of creeping around on their stomach or "scooting" (i.e., crawling on one leg and dragging the other or a combination of rocking, rolling, and squirming on their stomach, bottom, or back). They next move to the crawling position that defies the forces of gravity and enables them to rise to their hands and knees, which is the precursor of the crawling position by extending the arms and bending the knees when the head and neck are extended. The reflex is said to be incorporated when neurologic and muscular development allows independent limb movement for actual crawling.

While a dysfunction of the STNR may certainly indicate a neurological problem, their inappropriate responses are actually quite commonly seen in clinical practice, and their dysfunction can be reprogrammed with a coincident improvement in the neurological status of the host.

Overload/Underload (OU) Athletic Training

New ideas in Overload/Underload (OU) athletic training have recently emerged that are said to allow athletes to train more precisely for their sport. For example, in such training baseball pitchers are encouraged to practice throwing a baseball in an unnatural manner with their same side foot forward. They take the stance and throw "across their body" in an effort to build up certain muscles to enhance their performance. This movement pattern is inconsistent with predesignated human movement patterns. Their goal in such training is to increase an athlete's power, which they define as the rate at which one can perform work, or the ability to exert muscle force quickly. The proponents of these new techniques are quick to point out that the goal of increased performance is related to, but distinct from strength, which is defined as the ability to exert muscle force. In either case, these movement patterns have the potential to plasticize pathways that are pathological in the long run.

The advocates of OU training also claim that the mechanics are not affected if the tools used are not too heavy. However, this author believes that if the movement mechanics are already pathological, as described above, prior to starting these new exercises, these newer training techniques have a very high probability of plasticizing compromise. Further, it is this author's recommendation that no athlete venture into such neurologically sensitive movement patterns until those patterns that should be stable are, in fact, stable;

even then, these OU patterns hold great potential for neurological danger.

No matter how new and innovative these training techniques may seem, they have a high probability of being detrimental to optimal human performance because they encourage neurological dysfunction. Anaerobic and/or cross training, for example, done when there is an inadequate or unstable aerobic base can lead to overtraining and the myriad symptoms related to that syndrome. Further, by encouraging the human training with dysfunctional human movement patterns—generating voluntary movements contrary to the basic human fabric—can lead to degenerative changes later in life all for the immediate sake of the next trophy.

Functional Training

Functional training is the result of adequate exercise with appropriate recovery. The right exercises must be coupled with defined movement techniques in order to achieve the desired functional outcome. In most every case, functional neurologists are skilled to evaluate and treat these movement disorders and return the athlete to their sport in a better condition than most other therapies. This functional outcome is more than the ability to increase performance at a specific sport of event. Rather, it means maintaining the innate human movement patterns and building upon an intact neuraxis that performs according to its predesignated manner. This is functional training.

The Overtraining Syndrome

Appropriate conditioning requires a balance between increasing active demand and the use of remedial methods to improve skills or reverse environmental damage. However, the potential for overtraining is a very common finding in the functional neurological practice. Even the most elite athletes can be overtrained; it is a syndrome with specific signs and symptoms that appear when there is too much overload and too little recovery. Overtraining has a very high probability of causing both physical and psychological symptoms characteristic to the overtraining syndrome.

Overtraining happens when athletes train for competition or a specific event beyond their ability to recover. They often exercise longer and harder—they exceed their functional capacity—in order to improve. However, without adequate rest and recovery, these training programs can backfire, and performance actually suffers.

The Neurological Overtraining Syndrome

Besides functional overtraining there is neurological overtraining. Neurological overtraining is the concept that any exercise that exceeds the athlete's metabolic rate and/or functional capacity to perform useful work as defined by using manual muscle testing (MMT) as functional neurology is detrimental to the whole neuraxis and therefore to the structure, itself.

A neurological evaluation using fMMT is the key to both prevention and correction of the overtraining syndrome. A receptor-based evaluation of each different primitive reflex display may be the most powerful neurological tool for assessing overtraining in the earliest stage, and may provide the first objective sign, even before other symptoms appear. Such is the case with a dysfunctional TNR. Observing the first signs or subtlest clues of functional breakdown in an athlete's most primitive stages is critical to preventing further functional erosion. In order for this assessment to be effective, conducting a monthly receptor-based evaluation is very important.

Athletes who are persistently overtrained—those who continually reinforce movement patterns that are something other than human—generally fall short of their potential. Their level of human performance does not rise to their optimum because they ultimately train into their handicap. The rehabilitation of their possibilities may require 1) a reevaluation of their training goals and performance schedule, 2) reducing stress, 3) improving their nutrition, and 4) spend time rebuilding their aerobic and neurological bases. These athletes will each recover at their own rate, sometimes requiring six months to a year or two, before resuming effective competition.

Table 2: A COMPARISON BETWEEN THE ASYMMETRIC AND SYMMETRIC TONIC NECK REFLEXES		
Reflex	Posture	Response (Reaction)
Asymmetric Tonic Neck Reflex (ATNR)	Supine	Extension of the [†]UE/[‡]LEs on the side of head rotation; Flexion of the UE/LEs on the side opposite head rotation
Symmetric Tonic Neck Reflex (STNR)	Supine	With neck in flexion: Flexion synergy, which facilitates UE flexors and LE extensors; With neck in extension: Extension synergy, which facilitates UE extensors and LE flexors
[†]UE=Upper Extremity; [‡]LE=Lower Extremity		

Summary

With your patient on your table, check a flexor muscle and an extensor muscle on each side of their body. Now recheck each of these muscles relative to the patient turning their head turned to the right and to the left. Did you find a difference? That difference does not need to be relative to the appropriate display because there may be a functional difference that indicates the need for treatment. The point is that you just demonstrated the TNR display; muscles change relative to head rotation.

The TNR display does indeed persist beyond the toddler stage. It is an integral part of normal human movement and displays itself both functionally and dysfunctionally. The functional display encourages neurological and postural stability while the dysfunctional display means certain performance error.

A consciously healthy person is one who knows that practicing into their weakness brings detriment. Overtraining is a serious problem, yet it is one that can be successfully remedied. More importantly, it's easily prevented. A functional neurological examination has a very high probability of uncovering dysfunction and rehabilitating the movement before these newer exercises can be started.

While there may be considerable research that supports these new training techniques, none of the research takes into account the potential for prior functional neurological impairment. Further, a previously broken down movement pattern has a high probability of encouraging movement creations that were never intended for the human system. Unless and until more research is done that incorporates fMMT relative to primitive reflexes as a template for normal movement, it is this author's opinion that these ideas should be avoided at best and used with extreme caution at least.

Case Study #3

History and Presenting Complaints: Linda is a very fit 47 year old female athlete who had been having lower back pain for two weeks prior to this examination. It started after lots of bending, twisting, and reaching overhead to stock the shelves in her store. She had also been having some associated vague whole-head headaches and vertigo.

Exam Findings: During Linda's exam, both of her psoas major muscles appeared to be normally facilitated when using MMT to evaluate her lower extremities. However, relative to her ATNR, each psoas major appeared to display a functional facilitation on the side toward head rotation and functional inhibition on the side opposite head rotation. This display is opposite to that which would otherwise be expected, and therefore functionally pathological.

Imaging: A nine view cervical radiographic series indicated a reversal of Linda's cervical curve with an associated reduction in the disc space between C4 and C5, and C5 and C6, with a functional dyscoupling of her mid and distal cervical spine during right and left lateral bending.

Clinical Impression: Palpation of Linda's cervical spine confirmed the pathological spinal motion. There appeared to be inappropriate movement in the mid and lower cervical spine indicating the presence of muscle spasms that had a high probability of hindering the adequate propagation of primary afferents; a deafferentation syndrome.

Treatment Plan: The treatment involved the manual manipulation of the patient's upper and lower cervical spine in a coupled fashion in order to reestablish the functional juxtaposition of the involved vertebral segments.

Discussion: According to functional neurological principles, a bilateral psoas major dysfunction indicates the strong probability of an occipital fixation as opposed to a subluxation; the two findings are quite unique. Challenging the upper cervical spine and occiput as well as the cervicodorsal junctions and treating the findings accordingly brought about the expected psoas display relative to the TNR stimulation.

It is essential to realize that muscle performance is a functional display of the nervous system's CIS. Further, the CIS is an indication of the nervous system's readiness to respond, and it is predictable relative to what would be considered to be normal.

Receptor Based Solutions™
for Your Tonic Labyrinthine Reflex

*The Functional Display of Flexion
and Extension Synergies*

Introduction

Reciprocity is essential to the postural display relative to gravity. It is the ability to not only resist gravity but also to have functional movement while remaining upright. The tonic labyrinthine reflex (TLR) is one of the several functional inborn reflexes that monitor the position of the head in relation to gravity and allow humans to attain upright and stable posture.

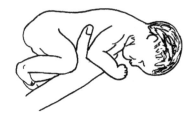

Figure 40: A flexion synergy

It is thought that the TLR arises at birth and gradually blends away anywhere from six weeks to three years later. The TLR is unique in that it arises from the labyrinth of the inner ear (the semicircular canals, utricles, and perhaps the saccules) and displays its preprogrammed response to gravity through the centerline structures creating various postures—primarily either a flexion or extension synergy (Figures 40 and 41, respectively), but it may also be related to side-lying, as right ear down or left ear down, and several other postures.

Recall that the semicircular canals are contained within the boney skull and serve a major function in the maintenance of equilibrium during movement. The utricular (and saccular) portion of the labyrinthine reflex appears to be concerned primarily with postural reflexes and in the differential distribution of muscle tone. Together, the particular stereotyped display of these TLRs is dependent upon both the postural (neuromuscular) position of the head on the neck and the head to its gravitational environment.

Synergistic Display

"Synergy" is the functional interaction between the several different elements in a system to produce an effect different from or greater than the sum of their individual effects. We see these functional interactions everywhere, ranging from the digestive flora that keeps

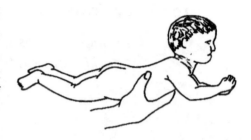

Figure 41: An extension synergy

our immune system at the ready to chemistry as with hydrogen and oxygen working together to make water, to cooperative interactions on an ant hill where order serves the queen. Synergy is a way of life in the physical world, including in the human body.

When we discuss neurologically functional synergies we mean the stereotypical movements that may be present and elicited in neurotypical individuals as well as in those with an atypical neurological display, but these characteristic movement patterns can also be provoked when encouraged during a functional neurological examination.

Functional Synergies

The functional flexion and extension synergies (Table 3) represent their unique and purposeful biases. In other words, while the muscles of balance are driven toward sodium equilibrium potential, or functional facilitation, the muscles of counterbalance are driven toward a potassium equilibrium potential, or functional inhibition, leading to the respective synergistic display. When a patient takes on a functional synergy, either a flexion synergy or an extension synergy, it manifests in stereotypical and atypical patterns across multiple joints. These are called *obligatory synergies* because they occur along homologous columns; they are hard wired into the human functional neurological program. They are described as either a flexion synergy or an extension synergy and affect both the upper and lower extremities.

Table 3: SYNERGISTIC DISPLAY IN THE EXTREMITIES		
Type of Synergy	**Upper Extremity**	**Lower Extremity**
Flexion Synergy	Scapular retraction and elevation, shoulder abduction and lateral rotation, elbow flexion, forearm supination, and wrist and finger flexion and adduction	Hip flexion, abduction and lateral rotation, knee flexion, ankle dorsiflexion and supination, and toe dorsiflexion
Extension Synergy	Scapular depression and protraction, shoulder medial rotation and adduction and internal rotation, elbow extension, forearm pronation, wrist extension, and finger flexion and adduction	Hip extension, adduction and medial rotation, knee extension, ankle plantar flexion and inversion, and toe plantar flexion and adduction
Note: Some muscles are not usually involved in these synergy patterns and include the latissimus dorsi, teres major, serratus anterior, finger extensors, and ankle evertors.		

When these synergies take on a dysfunctional pattern they tend to interfere with normal activities of daily living. Some aspects of the obligatory synergy patterns however, can be rehabilitated to increase function relative to the movement available to the individual. Obligatory synergy patterns can be evaluated by asking the patient to make certain voluntary movements, or as a result of stimulated reflexes.

For example, when a neurotypical person displays a flexion synergy, their structure takes on a characteristic posture where both upper and lower extremities and their torso have increased flexor tone relative to their extensor tone. Conversely, a neurotypical extensor synergy displays an increased extensor tone of all extremities and the torso relative to their flexor tone.

The neurotypical flexion and extension synergy postures are relatively simple to display. For example: Flexion of the head on the neck in the prone posture should cause an increased tone in the physiological flexors relative to the physiological extensors; it induces the fetal posture (Table 4). The body and extremities are driven more toward a flexion synergy when the CIS of the flexor muscles moves toward functional facilitation. This flexion display is demonstrated most prominently in the upper extremities, forearm, wrist, and fingers. It is demonstrated in the lower extremity as flexion of the hip, knee, supination of the ankle, and dorsiflexion of the ankles and toes.

Conversely, extending the head on the neck in the prone posture should cause an increased tone in the extensor muscles relative to the flexor muscles causing a stiffening of the back muscles, extension of the elbow, pronation of the forearm and extension of the wrist, and flexion and adduction of the fingers, with a concomitant straightening, stiffening, and pushing together of the legs, and the pointing of the toes. (Sometimes it is helpful to consider a running quadruped when considering these particular synergies.)

In the supine posture, there is a demonstrable functional facilitation of the extensors in all limbs and functional inhibition of all limb flexors.

The side lying posture induces a functional facilitation of the extensors of the limbs on the down side and a functional facilitation of the flexors on the up side, and a corresponding reciprocal functional inhibition of each of the antagonists.

An Important Blend of Reflexes

The TNR and TLR are functionally synergistic in their postural patterns. They are irrevocably and inseparably related in their purpose and their display. The TNR and TLR reinforce each other in their effects on the upper extremities and oppose each other in their effects on the lower extremities. The labyrinthine response alters muscle tone, extends, and changes the position of the upper limbs and head with the goal of supporting posture and maintaining balance of the body and head with respect to gravity.

These effects are modulated through the extrapyramidal components that involve the reticulospinal and vestibulospinal tracts, the latter reaching the spinal cord to terminate at cervical and upper thoracic levels.

The pontomedullary areas give rise to the medial (pontine) and lateral (medullary) reticulospinal pathways that act on the alpha and gamma motoneurons of the cord in order to modify and coordinate their particular reflexive displays. The medial reticulospinal tract is responsible for exciting anti-gravity, extensor muscles by facilitating extensor reflexes and inhibiting flexor responses while the lateral reticulospinal tract is involved with inhibiting excitatory axial extensor muscles of movement by inhibiting stretch reflexes in extensor muscles and facilitating flexor responses. The medial reticulospinal tract lends a modulatory influence to the lateral vestibulospinal tract related to problems of balance, although the vestibular pathways are more substantially involved. The reticulospinal tracts are also involved with the hypothalamic outflow that controls sympathetic thoracolumbar outflow and parasympathetic sacral outflow.

The medial and lateral vestibulospinal tracts originate in the lower portion of the pons and upper portion of the medulla. The medial vestibulospinal tract projects bilaterally from the medial vestibular nucleus within the medial longitudinal fasciculus to the ventral horns in the upper cervical cord (C6 vertebra). It promotes stabilization of head position by innervating the neck muscles, which helps with head coordination and eye movement. The lateral vestibulospinal tract is composed of fibers originating in the lateral, superior, and inferior vestibular nuclei (primarily the lateral). It runs down the total length of the spinal cord to provide excitatory signals to interneurons, which relay the signal to the motor neurons in antigravity muscles that facilitate extensors and inhibit flexors of the lower extremities in order to maintain upright and balanced postural mechanisms.

Signs of TLR Dysfunction

A functional TLR error most commonly appears as an extension or flexion synergy most commonly observed as problems with spatial recognition and visual perception, motion sickness, poor posture, and atypical muscle tone. The child may have difficulty lifting their head while lying supine and/or an inability to bring their hands together in the midline or overhead. When in the prone posture the child may demonstrate an excessive flexion with difficulty lifting their head to breathe.

Reflex	Posture	Response (Reaction)
Table 4: A COMPARISON OF THE FLEXION AND EXTENSION SYNERGIS SEEN IN THE TONIC LABYRINTHINE REFLEX DISPLAY		
Symmetric Tonic Labyrinthine Reflex	Prone with *flexion* of the head on the neck (similar display supine)	The body and extremities are held in a flexion synergy, most prominently seen in flexion of the elbow, and finger flexion and adduction, with a flexion of the hip and knee.
Symmetric Tonic Labyrinthine Reflex	Prone with *extension* of the head on the neck (similar display supine)	The body and extremities are held in an extension synergy, most prominently seen in shoulder adduction, forearm pronation, and finger flexion and adduction, with hip adduction, knee extension, and ankle plantar flexion.

Summary

Lay your patient supine and prone and check these postures. The intact nervous system should exhibit the preprogrammed posture with the appropriate facilitation and inhibition of the associated muscles. Any other muscle response should be considered pathological and deserves investigation.

It is important for the doctor to recognize these synergies and understand their implications in terms of neurotypical and pathological patterns. For example, the presence of an extension synergy in the muscles of the lower extremities (the hamstrings, for example) of a prone patient will tend to inhibit the patient's ability to resist the normal demands placed on these muscles during fMMTs.

According to the traditional medical reasoning, the presence of this dysfunctional primitive reflex together with others such as the ATNR past the first six months of life would have a very high probability of indicating developmental delay and/or neurological abnormalities, or when observed in the adult a potential CNS condition. Left uncorrected, the dysfunctional display may precipitate such a functional delay but it could also be avoided by normalizing the primitive reflex posture.

For example, in people with cerebral palsy, the reflexes may persist and even be more pronounced. As abnormal reflexes, both the TLR and the ATNR can cause problems for the growing child because they both tend to hinder functional activities such as rolling, crawling, bringing the hands together, or even bringing the hands to the mouth. Over time, both the TLR and ATNR can lead to more serious damage to the growing child's joints and bones, perhaps causing the head of the thigh bone to subluxate or, more seriously, dislocate altogether. However, another perspective might suggest a subluxated or fixated sacrum, or any other homologously related structural issue. These possibilities are just a few of those that should be considered when working with the TLR.

Case Study #4

History and Presenting Complaint: Cathy (56 year old female) presented with discomfort through her cervicodorsal spine, bilaterally, with associated bilateral numbness and tingling of her upper extremities. The symptoms were worse when lying in bed at any time of day and they would disappear when she was upright. As a result, she did not sleep well and felt unrefreshed when she woke.

Exam Findings: Her body temperature was 96.8F (oral); her heart rate was 76 beats per minute; her blood pressure was 110/60 bilaterally. Her height was 5'9" tall and she weighed 149 pounds. Her posture and gait were unremarkable.

The biceps, triceps, brachioradialis, patellar, and Achilles deep tendon reflexes all appeared to be +1 bilaterally. The gluteus maximus MMT appeared to be able to meet the demands of manual muscle testing bilaterally when in the prone posture, but a simultaneous extension of the patient's head on her neck appeared to induce a functional inhibition of the gluteus maximus bilaterally.

Imaging: A nine view radiographical series revealed a slight reversal of her cervical spine with a reduction of the disc space height between C5/6. There appeared to be a reversal of the AO mechanism with a concomitant +theta Y axial rotation of the atlas and a dyscoupling of the mid and distal cervical spine with right and left lateral bending. The neuroforamina all appeared to be widely patent bilaterally.

Clinical Impression: This patient displayed a dysfunctional tonic labyrinthine reflex in the prone posture.

Treatment Plan: Coupled palpation presented a fixation of the patient's upper cervical spine, which was reduced with normal coupled manual manipulation of the dysfunctional segments.

Response to Care: Follow up MMT of the gluteus maximus with the patient's head in neutral, flexion and extension indicated that, after treatment, the muscle was able to meet the demands that MMT placed upon it.

Discussion: The fixation of the upper cervical spinal motor segments appeared to have induced a functional inability of the gluteus maximus to perform according to its original design. Further, coupled manual manipulation of the upper cervical spine appeared to normalize the functional display, which reestablished appropriate stability in the gluteus maximus bilaterally.

Receptor Based Solutions™
for Your Flexor Withdrawal Reflex

A Physological Protective Response

Introduction

This chapter tackles the FWR/FRA to address its functional stimulation and display, and describe possible ways to effectively interpret and influence its flawed display.

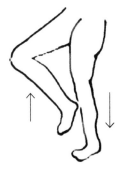

Figure 42: The Flexor Withdrawal Response of the lower extremities

The nociceptive or flexor withdrawal reflex (FWR; the sensory signal being a flexor reflex afferent, FRA) (Figure 42) is a cord-mediated reflex intended to protect the body from damaging stimuli. It is commonly used to assess the function of the nociceptive system despite the current lack of standardized stimulation procedures.

All human physiological reflexes have a predictable display. The classic example of the FWR is the reflexive withdrawal of an extremity when it is traumatized. Stepping on a tack (Figure 43) causes the predictable functional facilitation of physiological flexors and the concomitant functional inhibition of the physiological extensors in the troubled extremity. These physiological responses are well known; there are no other choices. The FWR either displays itself predictably or it is pathological. If a reflex displays itself in ways other than according to its originally preprogrammed format, that reflex should be considered "other-than-human," with a concomitantly increased risk of injury to the joint(s) involved. Reflex errors always require treatment and rehabilitation.

The FWR is a withdrawal from a noxious stimulus; a protective response. It quickly withdraws a traumatized body part away from perceived danger while maintaining posture and balance. It is impossible for any person to tell when their FWR has error because the response is reflexive. Further, it can be challenging to observe a dysfunctional FWR unless the observer knows what to anticipate.

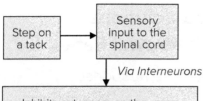

- Inhibits extensors on the same side
- Hip flexors facilitate on the same side; i.e., the leg lifts
- Extensors contract on the opposite side
- Inhibits flexors on the opposite side to maintain balance and support weight

Figure 43: A schematic of the Flexor Withdrawal Reflex

The sensory input synapses ipsilaterally in the spinal cord's gray matter and ultimately the anterior horn cells with a functional facilitation of the associated physiological flexors that cause withdrawal of the affected extremity from the stimulus, with a simultaneous and reciprocal response (through contralaterally synaptic pathways) of the contralateral extremity—a crossed cord reflex, which serves to enhance postural support during withdrawal of the affected limb from the painful stimulus, i.e., functional facilitation of the contralaterally associated physiological extensors, causing a pushing away from the stimulus.

Other interneurons instantaneously relay the sensory information up to the cerebellum, midbrain, basal ganglia, and cerebral cortex to integrate the nociceptive response and the consequential protective movement. However, the reflex's inappropriate display can lead to the realization of pain through various pathways.

A Babinski-Like Response

The FWR is a primitive withdrawal type response that is normal for the first few months of life and is thought to be suppressed by supraspinal activity sometime before six months of age. The FWR looks much like the Babinski reflex, but they are not the same. The Babinski response is the best known (and most important) of the so-called "pathological reflexes". The FWR is actually a superficial reflex that stimulates the same withdrawal display as the plantar or the Babinski reflex, but the FWR is not frankly pathological; it is physiologic. Therefore, we call the FWR *"Babinski-like."*

The full expression of the Babinski response upon scratching the sole of the foot from the heel along the lateral aspect of the sole and then across the ball of the foot to the base of the great toe (Figure 44) includes extension of the great toe and fanning of the other toes, which is thought to arise as a result of damage to the descending tracts from the brain that promotes a return of this primitive protective reflex while at the same time abolishing the normal plantar response.

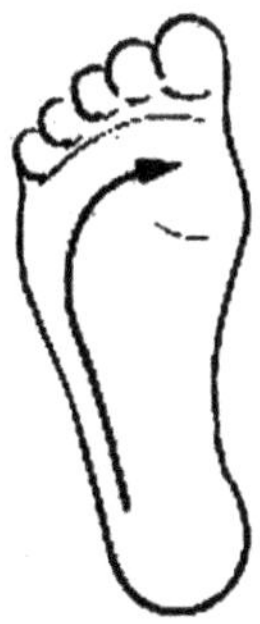

Figure 44: Elicit the Babinski-like reflex: scratch along the lateral aspect of the sole of the foot from the heel to the ball

The presence of a positive Babinski reflex in older children and adults indicates injury to the brain and spinal cord consistent with an upper motor neuron lesion. This same physiological response is also seen as a consequence of deafferentation in the more rostral aspects of the neuraxis that modifies the CIS of the centers that would have otherwise controlled such a response.

The FWR is said to be extinguished in the human system beyond about six months of age. However, despite that belief, it *is* clinically possible—and completely physiologically normal—to elicit the reflex's functional display when using fMMT as functional neurology. The normal plantar response is flexion of the great toe (i.e., a down-going toe) with a simultaneous flexion of the rest of the toes with a complementary withdrawal response of the foot.

Since we know the functional response, any other type of display must be considered pathological, leading to a dysfunctional afferent signal that causes a concomitant dysfunctional motor response.

Central Pattern Generator

Many reflex responses are housed in a network of neural connections called the central pattern generators (CPGs) that produce rhythmic functional outputs without sensory feedback; they are preprogrammed. For example, walking and swimming activities—and flying movements in birds—are largely controlled by the CPG for locomotion.

CPGs produce rhythmic outputs resembling normal "rhythmic motor patterns" even in isolation from motor and sensory feedback from limbs and other muscle targets. To be classified as a CPG, there must be two or more paths that intermingle such that each process sequentially increases and decreases. Further, as a result of this intermingling, the system repeatedly returns to its starting condition.

For example, like the CPGs, which act according to their own controls, the heart has its own intrinsic abilities. Taken out of the chest and set on a table, the heart's SA node—its inherent pacemaker—beats between 60–100 beats per minute. However, when connected to the functional influences of the autonomic system, the heart's normal rate is about 72 beats per minute. The brain's modulatory influence on the heart's rate influences its function. Similarly, but in a different manner, the CPG's are influenced by the CIS of the final common pathway.

Like the heart, the CPG's starting condition can physiologically drift relative to the CIS of anterior horn modulation. Recent evidence suggests that plastic changes can affect some CPG elements that may contribute to the development of specific dysfunctional conditions associated with compromised movement patterns or spontaneous movement disorders that mimic functional locomotion. The original CPG design remains fundamentally intact but its CIS drifts toward dysfunction.

Spinal Stepping Generator

The CPG that produces stepping behavior (the spinal stepping generator, SSG) is thought to be resident in the spinal cord. Although it is thought that the CPG is able to function independent of motor and sensory feedback from limbs and other muscle targets, that mechanism appears to be functionally influenced by the physiological effects of gait and posture at the anterior horn of the spinal cord. Receptor stimulation of the kind produced via the FWR should fortify the rhythmical activity attributed to that SSG. However, when the FWR exceeds the functional capacity that would otherwise maintain the usual intra- and intersegmental stepping patterns, the nervous system becomes functionally disorganized and begins to display movement patterns that are inconsistent with the original human spinal programming.

Functional limb movements are required for upright posture and meaningful gait (Table 5). This requires appropriately modulated internuncial networks that integrate centrifugal (descending) commands from the rostral neuraxis as well as those that are the result of functional input from segmental and centripetal (ascending) primary afferents. These modulatory effects are sensitive to the quality of reciprocated afferents from the periphery as well as the functional modulation of those controls that cascade through the basal ganglia and midbrain, brainstem, and cord, from cortical centers. Each of these disparate efferents must integrate in the anterior horn of the spinal cord

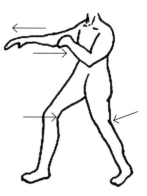

Figure 45: The Flexor Withdrawal Response of the upper and lower extremities

before meaningful movement can be induced. The *positive support phenomenon* is an integral part of this barrage; i.e., there must be functional reciprocity (Table 5) between antigravity muscles and those that would allow for purposeful movement.

The Upper Extremity Response

Similar to the lower extremity response is that of the upper (Figure 45) extremities. The classic example is the reflexive withdrawal of the offended part after touching a hot stove, for example, which will generate a reaction in the upper extremities much like, but contrary to, that of the lower extremities. The heat stimulates noxious receptors in the skin, triggering the primary afferents that travel to the spinal cord and then onward to all of its related synaptic connections, and also to the brain.

Specifically, nociceptive stimulation of the left upper extremity will cause its physiological withdrawal with a concomitant physiological extension—a pushing back—from the source of the noxious stimulation with the right upper extremity. This FWR of the upper extremity is displayed as a functional facilitation of the physiological flexors on the extremity of stimulation with a concomitant functional inhibition of the physiological extensors of that ipsilateral extremity, and the simultaneous functional facilitation of the physiological extensors on the upper extremity contralateral to stimulation with a concomitant functional inhibition of the physiological flexors of that extremity.

Stimulus \ Response ↓ →	Ipsilateral Upper Extremity	Contralateral Upper Extremity	Ipsilateral Lower Extremity	Contralateral Lower Extremity
Stroke palm of hand	Facilitates physiological flexors and inhibits physiological extensors	Facilitates physiological extensors and inhibits physiological flexors	Facilitates physiological extensors and inhibits physiological flexors	Facilitates physiological flexors and inhibits physiological extensors
Stroke sole of foot	Facilitates physiological extensors and inhibits physiological flexors	Facilitates physiological flexors and inhibits physiological extensors	Facilitates physiological flexors and inhibits physiological extensors	Facilitates physiological extensors and inhibits physiological flexors

Table 5: FUNCTIONAL RECIPROCITY AND THE FLEXOR WITHDRAWAL REFLEX

The Flexor Reflex Afferent and Autonomic Concomitants

It is of upmost importance to remember that for every primary afferent that reaches the spinal cord there are a dozen associated neurological events that take place inside the cord (Table 1). Each of these events has its individual effect on the neuraxis both segmentally and rostrally according to its relationships, and together these 12 events express themselves in preprogrammed patterns of movement that are uniquely human. The various options provide for a myriad display that can adapt and change to the internal and external environment stimuli as needed. However, any and/or every individual or global timing error will have its consequence at some level of involvement and it is the doctor's challenge to find and fix these errors and return the patient to their normal display.

Two Very Important Clinical Notes

First, when stimulating the FRA, the clinician has about 4-5 seconds to examine the response because of the way the FRA decays in the cord. It deteriorates relatively slowly in order to both maintain the withdrawal, and facilitate balance and stance to prevent a fall.

Second, any FRA supersedes any other FRA independent of their timing. Again, this is protective. As a result, when testing the FRA stimulus or FWR display, any extremity can be examined and the tests can be repeated relatively quickly without concern for cord bias.

Summary

The FWR is the manifestation of a nociceptive (a provocation with the potential to do damage) stimulus. As a result, the limb protects itself and the rest of the body—a survival response—by withdrawal. This FWR is always at the root of neurological performance but it does not always display itself according to its original programming.

Consider that again: The normal lower extremity response to a noxious stimulus, such as stroking the sole of the foot with a sharp object, should cause a physiological withdrawal of the ipsilateral lower extremity and physiological extension of the contralateral lower extremity, increasing the resistance to fall. The upper extremity response is the same process as the lower extremity, but reciprocal as described in the Table 4, above.

Adaptive change can cause the slow migration of an anticipated response to a pathological one that is not according to the preprogrammed human pattern. This dysfunction deserves investigation and treatment in order to return its function to what is considered to be neurotypical.

Case Study #5

History and Presenting Complaints: Michael (male, 54yo) came in complaining of twitching in his left hip for the past three to four days. He had no idea how the twitching started, but said he had been under a lot of personal and professional stress the past two weeks.

Examination Findings: One aspect of Michael's examination indicated that stroking the sole of either foot with a sharp object caused the inhibition of the proximal rectus femoris ipsilaterally with an erroneous facilitation of the proximal rectus femoris contralaterally; this is opposite of what one would expect, both ipsilaterally and contralaterally.

The clinical impression of the entire neurological examination indicated that Michael was deafferentated through his cervicodorsal spine and left shoulder girdle, and he was not ventilating properly, affecting his left cerebellum.

Imaging: A seven view lumbar series appeared to show a loss of the lumbar lordotic curve with a concomitant dyscoupling upon lateral bending right and left, and a reduction in the L5/S1 disc space.

Clinical Impression: According to Michael's original diagnosis, increasing the afferentation to his left cerebellum would have a high probability of normalizing his FWR.

Treatment: Coupled chiropractic manual manipulation of Michael's left cervicodorsal spine and left shoulder girdle together with certain specific physiological exercises to rehabilitate his structure and nervous system in order to normalize his FWR.

Response to Care: Subsequently, stroking the sole of his foot with a sharp object caused the proper physiological response—the functional facilitation of the proximal ipsilateral rectus femoris and contralateral hamstrings, and the functional inhibition of the proximal rectus femoris contralaterally and hamstrings ipsilaterally. This response is more human-like.

Discussion: (In this clinical case, we will only focus on the lower extremity's response to nociception, but there is also an upper body response.) As a result of noxious stimulation, one would expect physiological withdrawal on the side of stimulation and positive support to resist falling down, contralaterally. That is, we would expect to observe physiological flexion of the thigh on the hip ipsilateral to stimulation and physiological extension of the thigh on the hip contralateral to that same type of stimulation.

This patient's erroneous FWR display is significant. It suggests that a painful (nociceptive) stimulus to either of Michael's feet might (figuratively) cause him to collapse onto the stimulus (discussed in the "Spinal Pattern Generator" videos, available from HealthBuilderS® Publishing). The examination indicated that his nervous system was originally unable to update fast enough to maintain upright posture. Actually, if Michael were to receive a stimulus that was significant enough to impact his capacity for upright posture, his lower body flexors would functionally inhibit increasing his probability of falling. Michael received other therapies to functionally rehabilitate his flexor withdrawal responses and left the office able to respond nominally.

Receptor Based Solutions™ for Your Galant Reflex

The Postural Response to Stroking the Lumbar Flank

Introduction

The Galant reflex (GR) (Figure 46), also known as the Spinal Galant Reflex, (SGR) or Galant's infantile reflex, is named after the Russian neurologist Johann Susman Galant. In his 1917 doctoral dissertation, Galant apparently believed the reflex to be a deep abdominal reflex in newborns, involving the contraction of the abdominal muscles upon tapping the anterior superior iliac spine or touching the skin along the spine from the shoulder to the hip. However, the literature seems to have abandoned the original deep abdominal response in favor of its being largely classified as a superficial reflex.

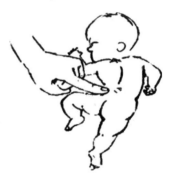

It is commonly taught that the Galant reflex is physiologically present during infancy until about the sixth month, being

Figure 46: The Galant Reflex

always pathological at higher ages. Further, the literature appears to imply that the GR causes the facilitation of the proximal ipsilateral quadriceps. However, over time, the ideas about GR seem to have changed.

The Superficial Reflex

A discussion of superficial reflex display must precede any analysis of the Galant or flexor withdrawal reflexes.

The superficial reflex described as stroking or scratching the skin was apparently first described by Rosenbach, in 1876, when he observed contractions of abdominal musculature induced by gentle scratching of the skin. This response has become commonly termed a superficial abdominal reflex, although considerable doubt exists concerning the superficial reflex's basic mechanisms.

Since Galant's reflex can be provoked by stroking the skin along the spine from the shoulder to the hip, it is a type of superficial reflex rather than a deep tendon reflex. While a functional deep tendon reflex is elicited by a sharp tap on the appropriate tendon or muscle to induce a brief stretch of the muscle followed by its contraction, the superficial reflex is any withdrawal reflex elicited by noxious or tactile stimulation.

Any withdrawal reflex elicited by noxious or tactile stimulation of the skin, cornea, or mucous membrane, including the corneal reflex, pharyngeal reflex, cremasteric reflex, etc., is a superficial reflex. Such superficial reflexes are the motor response to scraping of the skin over various areas, classically over the abdomen to observe an umbilical response, the inner thigh for the cremasteric response, or the anus to display the "anal wink."

The abdominal reflex displays as the contraction of the abdominal muscles in the proximity of the abdomen that is roused by scraping the skin of the abdomen around the umbilicus. This contraction can often be seen as an abrupt motion of the umbilicus toward the area that is stimulated. The cremaster reflex should produce a brisk and brief elevation of the testicle on that side. The "anal wink" is a contraction of the external anal sphincter when the skin near the anal opening is scratched. This and other superficial reflexes are often abolished in spinal cord damage.

Other superficial reflexes are the plantar (or flexor withdrawal) reflex, the Galant, and the new Modified and Upper Galant reflexes.

The superficial reflex is rated simply relative to its presence or absence, although any deviation from that which is an anticipated response should be considered abnormal, or pathological. While superficial reflex testing is mandatory when there is suspicion of an upper motor neuron lesion, their abnormal response is often clinically the result of a mismatch between the receptor and the spinal cord. If the superficial reflex is absent and the deep tendon reflex is increased, this will add evidence to indicate an upper motor neuron lesion and reason for consultation for neurodiagnostic testing.

An important distinction between deep tendon and superficial reflexes is that the former reflex will be amplified when the patient is distracted, whereas the latter reflex will not change. In each case the reflexes will be absent in the presence of a central or peripheral condition, and that condition can relate to a neurophysiological lesion secondary to a deafferentation syndrome. While these reflexes may be depressed or absent in patients with functional lesions in the more rostral CNS, they can also display an abnormal response using fMMT as functional neurology.

The Galant Reflex Display

The GR is commonly tested in newborns to help rule out brain damage at birth and is said to fade between the ages of four and six months of age. The GR is thought to be important in the development of hearing and auditory processing, as well as helping to achieve balance when the child is creeping and crawling.

Classically, one would elicit the GR by holding the newborn in a face down posture (either with the baby's stomach in the examiner's hand) or laying them on their stomach and stroking the skin along the one side of the lumbar spine. The normal reaction is for a responsive baby to rotate or flex the hips and body toward the stroked side. It has been thought that this reaction involves the concomitant functional facilitation of the ipsilateral quadriceps (Figure 46) and a simultaneous functional inhibition of the ipsilateral hamstrings, eventually—it has been reported—helping the baby turn onto its back as their nervous system matures.

The common belief is that a persistent GR response beyond six months of age is a pathological sign. Literature teaches that a retained GR can lead to a child's inability to control their bladder, which may involve bedwetting issues at a later age. Further, the child may be unable to sit still for any period and/or they might fidget when wearing waistbands that are too tight, or from tags in clothing; apparently, even the back of a chair can activate the reflex. The reflex is also said to have a great impact on attention and concentration, which also affects the short term memory because of an incessant need to be in constant motion.

Galant and the *f*MMT

The functional use of this GR, however, demonstrates this series of beliefs to be unfortunate. This author believes in the importance of the GR's integration with the rest of the functional reflexes and has observed a concomitant functional involvement of the ipsilateral hamstrings. As a result, there is fundamental disagreement regarding the unfortunate assertion of both the GR's disappearance and pathogenicity. While the general belief holds the GR to be pathological if it persists beyond six months of age, clinical experience has demonstrated that the GR is an integral part of every human being's ability to attain an upright posture, and it can be demonstrated in every patient no matter their age, and its specifically pathological finding being its dysfunctional display relative to *f*MMT.

In reality, regular *f*MMT testifies to the fact that the GR *should* persist. The GR is essential to the reciprocal integration of centerline antigravity muscles and their physiological integration with the functional neurological matrix that eventually enables upright posture and it can be demonstrated in patients at any age. It is the GR's dysfunctional display that is clinically important. One example, among many, is the involvement of spinal dysfunction with bladder pathology via the vesico-sympathetic, vesico-parasympathetic and vesico-pudendal reflexes.

This author has regularly used *f*MMT to test the hamstrings as a group and found that a previously functionally facilitated hamstring will become functionally inhibited after stroking the ipsilateral lumbar flank (Table 6) in a rostral to caudal direction, indicating some sort of superficial reflex response related to the lumbar area. Further, it has been found that—while the patient is in a prone posture—reaching underneath to the patient's abdomen and stroking the skin lateral to the umbilicus in a medial to lateral direction with a sharp object displays the same functional inhibitory response in the ipsilateral hamstring.

Be careful when stimulating the superficial reflex to not create a significant noxious stimulus that leads to a guarding or withdrawal response rather than a reflexive display.

Three Galant Reflexes

The Galant, Modified Galant, and Upper Galant reflexes participate in attaining purposeful upright posture, otherwise known as the tonic lumbar reflex in the more matured nervous system.

As a result of the previously described physiological lateral deviation or flexion of the hips toward the side of the paraspinal stimulation, the dysfunctional GR, MGR, and/or UGR can generate an odd posture or odd balance in walking or running secondary to the chronic and uncorrected involuntary body twisting or pivoting with autonomic concomitants consistent with their own unique physiological bias.

Table 6: FUNCTIONAL RECIPROCITY OF THE GALANT REFLEX IN RESPONSE TO STROKING THE LUMBAR FLANK*		
Stimulus \ Response ↓ →	Ipsilateral Hamstring	Contralateral Hamstring
Stroke Lateral to the Lumbar Spine	Inhibition	Facilitation
*More information on the GR and the Modified Galant reflex (MGR) can be found in, "Cortical release signs: the modified Galant reflex using applied kinesiology as functional neurology."		

Summary

It was originally thought that a child's normal neurological maturation should cause the GR extinction by the fourth to sixth month of age, but now we learn the GR is a vital part of all functional neurological testing no matter the patient's age.

Demonstrate the reflex for yourself. Lay your patient on your table prone and check a hamstring muscle for its integrity. Note your findings, then stroke the lateral portion of their ipsilateral lumbar spine with your thumb nail and immediately retest the ipsilateral hamstring. Did its integrity change? The normal finding is for the inhibition of hamstring ipsilateral to the stroked lumbar flank. Both the functional facilitation of a previously functionally inhibited hamstring and/or the functional inhibition of a previously functionally facilitated hamstring indicate the need for further evaluation.

While the GR is generally considered to an essential test to evaluate the presence of an upper motor neuron lesion, its dysfunctional presence may also be related to a dysfunctional response to upright posture and gravity. Always keep the more serious pathology in mind during your investigation and recheck your findings often. A resolution of the dysfunctional finding is a good thing for the patient but, as with any of these functional reflexes, if the condition persists then the referral to a specialist is appropriate.

Case Study #6

History and Presenting Complaint: Kelly (37 year old female) has been a patient for a long period. She recently came in complaining of lower back pain along her lumbosacral spine and sacroiliac joints bilaterally, with that of the left side being more involved than that of the right, for the past two weeks. She had been doing a lot of bending and twisting to unpack boxes after her move, but she felt no specific incident that would create such pain. There appeared to be no other significant history.

Examination: As a small part of the entire physical examination, which included *f*MMT, the patient was placed in a prone posture. Examination of the lower extremity appeared to show that the hamstrings were able to meet the demands of *f*MMT bilaterally. Further, tapping the tendons of the origin and insertion of the ipsilateral medial hamstring caused appropriate functional facilitation of that hamstring.

Stroking the skin over the distal paraspinal muscles on either side from the dorsolumbar spine to the sacroiliac joint with a sharp object (as if to stimulate the GR), appeared to cause a functional facilitation of the ipsilateral hamstring (Table 5).

Imaging: Seven views of the lumbar spine appeared to show a reduction of the normal lumbar lordosis with a concomitant dyscoupling of the mid and lower lumbar spine with both right and left lateral deviation. There appeared to be some generalized eburnation of the lumbar facets bilaterally, more distally than rostrally. The L5/S1 disc space showed only a mild reduction in size.

Treatment Plan: A sacral challenge revealed the need for its coupled structural manipulation. Subsequent reevaluation of Kelly's GR indicated a normal response—functional inhibition of the hamstrings ipsilaterally and functional facilitation of the hamstrings contralaterally. Further, nociceptive stimulation to the sole of the patient's foot appeared to indicate a nominal flexor withdrawal response bilaterally.

Response to Care: Reevaluation of the hamstring response to *f*MMT indicated a predictable response, bilaterally.

Discussion: The appropriate GR display appears to possibly involve the functional facilitation of the ipsilateral quadriceps. Therefore, the reciprocal response should cause inhibition of the ipsilateral hamstrings.

One general rule in applied kinesiology is that the bilateral involvement of a muscle indicates a possible spinal fixation, and each muscle involvement indicates a particular level of the fixation. For example, a bilateral hamstring involvement suggests a possible sacral fixation. In Kelly's case, the hamstrings appear to be functionally facilitated when tested individually, with a concomitant dysfunctional facilitation relative to the functional facilitation of the ipsilateral quadriceps secondary to nociceptive stimulation via the GR; a pathological display.

Summary: This patient is a neurotypical 37 year old female. She had no frank brain pathology but there was some demonstrable dysfunctional reflexive display with concomitant uncoupled spinal involvement. The GR showed itself to be a valuable part of her functional neurological examination. It revealed the functional sacral instability, with treatment bringing about the proper resolution of that dysfunction. The GR should be a fundamental part of every patient's neurological examination, despite their age.

Receptor Based Solutions™
for Your Crossed Extensor Reflex

The Importance of Reciprocity to Human Performance

Introduction

Consider the moment of a reflexive response: A reflex is a series of swift and pre-loaded movement patterns that occur in response to some sort of stimulus applied to the periphery and transmitted centrally—to the spinal cord (Figure 47) and/or brain—before one even realize they are responding to it.

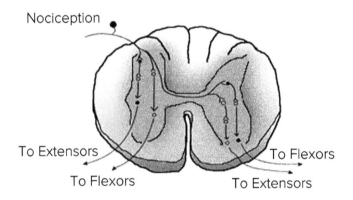

Nociception

To Extensors

To Flexors

To Flexors

To Extensors

Figure 47: A cross section through the spinal cord

The Crossed Extensor Reflex (CER) is a reciprocal response, generally considered protective. It is related to both the deep tendon and flexor withdrawal reflexes through the activity in the gray matter of the cord in response to some stimulus, often nociceptive. The sensory impulses that convey some sort of neurological insult (nociception) travel at about 0.5 meters (less than two feet) per second. Conversely, those sensory impulses that convey joint position sense (proprioceptors) travel faster than the length of a football field (120 meters; almost 400 feet) in one second.

Protective Response

The CER is basically a withdrawal reflex on one side of the body with the addition of certain inhibitory pathways needed to maintain balance and coordination. Therefore, when a potentially injurious stimulus occurs, the protective reflex response of moving away from that threat happens much faster than the conscious recognition of the impending insult.

Nociception is always present; everyone has it. However, nociception is kept under control by many factors. Joint motion, chemical signals, hormones, etc., all stifle nociception until something disrupts their modulatory controls. It is only then that nociception is allowed to reach conscious levels and one realizes pain.

The CER is another example of a protective response, that apparently begins at about 28 weeks gestation and is said to be neurologically integrated one to two months after birth. It is functionally significant in reciprocal muscle actions. Its dysfunction can interfere with activities like running and kicking, and other purposeful events.

Of the cord's 12 responses to one primary afferent, eight of them have to do with muscles. This means that three quarters (75 percent) of the spinal cord responses to incoming signals have to do with reciprocal muscle function.

The CER response intimately links the deep tendon reflex (DTR) with the flexor withdrawal response (FWR). Where stimulating the patellar tendon with a fast stretch causes functional facilitation of the ipsilateral rectus femoris, for example, the normal CER display functionally inhibits the hamstring ipsilaterally (Table 7).

Table 7: FUNCTIONAL RECIPROCITY OF THE PATELLAR DEEP TENDON AND CROSS CORD REFLEXES		
Muscle \ Reflex ↓ →	If the Patellar DTR is Stimulated Ipsilaterally, then...	If the Patellar DTR is Stimulated Contralaterally, then...
Rectus femoris	Facilitated at its insertion	Inhibited at its insertion
Hamstring	Inhibited at its insertion	Facilitated at its insertion

While both the CER and FWR are protective, the CER expresses the reciprocal activity of the FWR (Table 8), i.e., when the FWR occurs, the flexors in the withdrawing limb contract and the extensors relax while the opposite occurs contralaterally. Where stroking the sole of one foot with a sharp object causes the physiological withdrawal of the ipsilateral foot from the stimulus, the reciprocal CER response causes physiological extension of the contralateral leg. That is, the stimulus causes functional facilitation of the proximal aspect of the ipsilateral rectus femoris; it also causes the functional inhibition of the proximal aspect of the ipsilateral hamstrings and proximal aspect of the contralateral rectus femoris with a simultaneous facilitation of the proximal aspect of the contralateral hamstrings.

Table 8: FUNCTIONAL CROSS-CORD RECIPROCITY AND THE FLEXOR WITHDRAWAL REFLEX		
Stimulus \ Response ↓ ➝	Ipsilaterally	Contralaterally
Stroke palm of hand	Facilitates upper extremity physiological flexors and inhibits physiological extensors	Inhibits upper extremity physiological flexors and facilitates physiological extensors
Stroke palm of hand	Inhibits lower extremity physiological flexors and facilitates physiological extensors	Facilitates lower extremity physiological flexors and inhibits physiological extensors
Stroke sole of foot	Facilitates lower extremity physiological flexors and inhibits physiological extensors	Inhibits lower extremity physiological flexors and facilitates physiological extensors
Stroke sole of foot	Inhibits upper extremity physiological flexors and facilitates physiological extensors	Facilitates upper extremity physiological flexors and inhibits physiological extensors

A good example of the protective nature of the CER is stepping on a tack. Staying consistent with the above example, consider that the tack pierced the person's left foot. The nociception-filled left foot reflexively pulls away from the noxious stimulus while the right leg sustains the weight of the whole body.

Here is the reflex: In general, the nociception causes physiological facilitation of the ipsilateral proximal rectus femoris (and other quadriceps muscles) while that ipsilateral proximal hamstring gets physiologically inhibited, allowing the thigh to flex on the hip. Simultaneously, the ipsilateral distal rectus femoris physiologically inhibits whereas the ipsilateral distal hamstrings—the semimembranosus, semitendinosus, and biceps femorus—physiologically facilitate, causing the left lower extremity to flex at the hip and knee. Meanwhile, the CER causes physiological facilitation of the right proximal hamstrings at the hip and physiological inhibition at the knee while that ipsilateral rectus femoris (and other quadriceps muscles) physiologically facilitates at its distal aspect and physiologically inhibits at its proximal aspect, thereby causing the right lower extremity to underpin the resistance to gravity.

Another example of a CER is touching a hot stove with the hand. As we saw in the FWR article, the irritated hand aggressively pulls away from the stimulus while the other hand quickly extends to push away from the stimulus. On the affected side, the arm physiologically flexes at the shoulder and elbow while the reciprocal happens contralaterally; there is physiological extension at the shoulder and elbow. Further, the protection also involves the lower extremities causing a step backward with the leg ipsilateral to the stimulus.

Summary

Both the FWR and CER are practically one and the same reflex. Where the FWR describes an extremity's response to a potentially dangerous stimulus, the CER describes the protective response of the rest of the body. When considered together, much can be learned about the functional state of the lower extremity reflexes relative to themselves as well as how these lower extremity reflexes relate to those of the upper extremities, and vice versa. The treatment varies relative to the site of the lesion, the discovery of which is the art of the functional application.

Case Study #7

History and Presenting Complaint: Adam (male, 23yo) was experiencing shooting pain through his left hip as far as his gluteal fold. It happened when he stepped wrong on his left foot and turned his ankle about two weeks prior to his visit.

Examination Findings: We performed the usual functional neurological examination. Relative to his feet, stroking the sole of Adam's right foot with a sharp object caused the nominal lower extremity functional response both ipsilaterally and contralaterally. Conversely, stroking the sole of his left foot with a sharp object caused functional facilitation of his ipsilateral rectus femoris and hamstrings, with a concomitant functional facilitation of the hamstrings and functional inhibition of the rectus femoris, contralaterally.

Imaging: Seven views of the patient's lumbar spine were obtained, which appeared to show a slight right lateral displacement of the lumbar spine with a concomitant reduction in the lumbar lordosis. There appeared to be a dyscoupling of the lumbar spine with right and left lateral bending and an eburnation of the lumbar facets more distally than rostrally, bilaterally. There appeared to be a slight reduction of the lumbosacral disc space. Otherwise all other soft tissues appeared to be unremarkable as far as they were visualized.

Clinical Impression: It is quite possible that the nociceptive FRA was stimulated each time the patient stepped on his left foot with a concomitant pathological facilitation of his hamstrings ipsilaterally. Over time, this dysfunction has the possibility of contributing to ipsilateral lower extremity involvement and other postural troubles.

Treatment: In this case, manipulation of the left talocalcaneal joint reset Adam's dysfunctional CER and his pain immediately ceased. A recheck of the lower extremity CER showed its response to be as anticipated, bilaterally.

Response to Care: The patient responded well to the care given with an increased functional display in his lower extremities.

Discussion: It appears that while the left rectus femoris, and the right rectus femoris and hamstrings were responding as expected, the left hamstrings displayed a pathological response. Since inappropriate joint motion leads to the experience of pain, this finding had a high probability of being related to Adam's experience of pain.

Adam's functional neurological response to the repetitive nociception revealed an excellent example of how a dysfunctional FWR generates a concomitant CER that may or may not be pathological. In this case, the FWR display contralateral to stroking the right foot was appropriate, the pathological response remaining within the left lower extremity when sole of the foot was stroked ipsilaterally.

With each step, the subluxation generated dysfunctional primary afferents from the left ankle leading to an inability to functionally inhibit the nociceptive reflexogenic afferents in the dorsal cord, leading to Adam's perception of pain in the area of the ipsilateral proximal hamstrings.

Receptor Based Solutions™ for Your Upper Galant Response

An Original Postural Response to Stroking and Tapping the Upper and Lower Back

Introduction

Daily practice is never dull when using functional reflexes. New ideas tend to spring up at the most opportune times and many of them are clinically relevant. Considering the value of the Galant and Modified Galant reflexes and their common usage relative to the newer findings in other chapters, the idea occurred to this author that perhaps there was a way to use them to gain more information relative to the upper body; to understand more about the ventral and dorsal spinocerebellar, cuneocerebellar, and spinothalamic pathways. One such new application is the Upper Galant Reflex (UGR) (Figure 48). It can be tested using the deltoid and clavicular portion of the pectoralis major muscles (PMC), but any other combination can be used, too.

Postural Change and Functional Display

We have previously discussed the effects of postural change on reflexive display. Patients do not live their lives in just one posture. Their postures constantly change, so check them from a supine to a prone posture, turn the head one way or the other, or stroke one foot relative to the other. Constantly evaluate the *f*MMT display. It is also useful to check patients in various postures to further understand the patient's functional signs and symptoms and formulate an effective treatment program.

The GR and MGR examination procedures are both described in the prone posture, but these new applications provide a greater understanding of the same stimuli in the seated and upright postures.

This new and exciting revelation allows for greater application of cerebellar and thalamic afferents and the ability for the patient's nervous system to attain upright posture.

Advanced Galant Application

Previous chapters in this series have explained GR and MGR tests using the hamstring and quadriceps muscles during fMMT. This UGR procedure uses the deltoid and the PMC muscles bilaterally to evaluate the physiological response to both stroking and tapping the upper and lower back relative to the upright posture (Table 9)— both seated and standing; the same techniques can also be done supine or prone. The technique of eliciting the Galant-like response is otherwise relatively unchanged aside from the patient's postural orientation to gravity and the fMMT being applied.

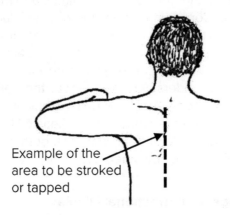

Example of the area to be stroked or tapped

Figure 48: The Upper Galant Reflex test

Relative to the ipsilateral deltoid findings insofar as stroking the upper dorsal spine is concerned, the UGR display is much like that of original GR test relative to the ipsilateral hamstrings after stroking lateral to the ipsilateral lumbar spine (Table 10). That is, *stroking the area closest to the deltoid or hamstrings causes the functional inhibition of that related muscle.* If the examiner keeps this one basic concept in mind and understands the general nuances of both the GR and UGR tests, applying these tests should become second nature.

Table 9: FUNCTIONAL RECIPROCITY OF THE UPPER GALANT REFLEX IN RESPONSE TO TESTING THE CLAVICULAR DIVISION OF THE PECTORALIS MAJOR (PMC) AND DELTOID MUSCLES AFTER STROKING OR TAPPING ALONG THE SPINE				
Stimulation\Response ↓ →	Ipsilateral PMC	Contralateral PMC	Ipsilateral Deltoid	Contralateral Deltoid
Stroke Lateral to the Upper Thoracic Spine (Above T6)	Facilitation	Inhibition	Inhibition	Facilitation
Tap Lateral to the Upper Thoracic Spine (Above T6)	Inhibition	Facilitation	Facilitation	Inhibition
Stroke Lateral to Lumbar Spine (Below T6)	Inhibition	Facilitation	Facilitation	Inhibition
Tap Lateral to Lumbar Spine (Below T6)	Facilitation	Inhibition	Inhibition	Facilitation

Special Note: Both the ipsilateral and contralateral responses of the PMC to both stroking and tapping with the UGR are similar to that of the GR, using the hamstrings.

Table 10: FUNCTIONAL RECIPROCITY OF THE UPPER GALANT REFLEX IN RESPONSE TO TESTING THE HAMSTRING AND DELTOID MUSCLES AFTER STROKING OR TAPPING ALONG THE SPINE				
Stimulation\Response ↓ →	Ipsilateral Hamstring	Contralateral Hamstring	Ipsilateral Deltoid	Contralateral Deltoid
Stroke Lateral to the Upper Thoracic Spine (Above T6)	Facilitation	Inhibition	Inhibition	Facilitation
Tap Lateral to the Upper Thoracic Spine (Above T6)	Inhibition	Facilitation	Facilitation	Inhibition
Stroke Lateral to Lumbar Spine (Below T6)	Inhibition	Facilitation	Facilitation	Inhibition
Tap Lateral to Lumbar Spine (Below T6)	Facilitation	Inhibition	Inhibition	Facilitation

Special Note: Both the ipsilateral and contralateral responses of the deltoid muscle to both stroking and tapping with the UGR are opposite to that of the GR, using the hamstrings.

Summary

The UGR is a novel and appropriate application of the same procedures used with the GR and MGR. It is a valuable adjunct to every neurological examination. As we have discussed with other functional reflexes, put your patient on your table and check these reflexes. Demonstrate for yourself that they do persist and that they are useful in both diagnosis and reevaluation of treatment.

Where the GR and MGR are commonly elicited with the patient in the prone posture each can also be easily stimulated with the patient in the seated and upright posture, too. These tapping and stroking stimuli of the lower body generally rise to the more rostral neuraxis via the ventral spinocerebellar and spinothalamic tracts, respectively. Further, since the UGR relates to stimulation rostral to T6, the cerebellar afferents are uniquely from the dorsal spinocerebellar and cuneocerebellar pathways with their distinctive cerebellar concomitants while the spinothalamic input is unchanged.

Case Study #8

History and Presenting Complaint: Jim (male 42yo) has been a patient for about six months. He originally presented with the complaint of twitching through his posterior upper back bilaterally with associated twitching through his left upper extremity. He has been previously diagnosed with a chronic degenerative condition that requires regular treatment.

Examination: The original examination findings included a litany of primitive reflex dysfunctions, all of which favorably respond to care but his degenerative condition requires constant remedial work. For the purposes of this UGR, the left deltoid examination indicated a functional inhibition without functional facilitation upon tapping the upper dorsal spine ipsilaterally or lumbar spine contralaterally, or when stroking the upper dorsal spine contralaterally or lumbar spine ipsilaterally. Further, the left PMC demonstrated a functional facilitation without functional inhibition upon tapping the ipsilateral upper dorsal spine or contralateral lumbar spine, or with stroking the contralateral upper dorsal spine or contralateral lumbar spine.

Imaging: Nine views of the patient's cervical spine appeared to show a slight reversal of the normal cervical lordosis with a concomitant reduction in the disc space height between C4/5 and C5/6 with a posterior displacement of C4 upon C5 seen in the neutral lateral view. That displacement appears to normalize in the flexion view and exaggerate in the extension view. There appeared to be dyscoupling of the mid and distal cervical spine with both right and left lateral bending. The neuroforamina all appeared to be widely patent bilaterally and all soft tissues appeared to be unremarkable as far as they were visualized.

Clinical Impression: It appears that this patient experiences a flexion synergy of the left upper body flexors with a concomitant functional inhibition of the left upper body extensors. This clinical picture appears to indicate a possible pyramidal display in the upper body on the left, which requires further evaluation and careful treatment.

Treatment: The patient has been treated with coupled manual manipulation of his right sternoclavicular articulation as well as his cervicodorsal spine and other spinal-related segments to reduce the apparent pyramidal distribution of weakness. He has been given certain complex movement therapies for his right upper and lower extremities and linear movement therapies for his left upper and lower extremities to enhance cerebellar balance. Further, he was instructed in certain specific exercises to enrich his left cortical integrity and enhance its appropriate outflow.

Response to Care: During the course of care there is constant discussion relative to the persistent degenerative condition. His familiar twitching persists, but its intensity and frequency have been greatly reduced.

Discussion: The functional inhibition of the left deltoid with a concomitant functional facilitation of the left PMC encourages the further examination of the cerebellar afferents from the dorsal and cuneocerebellar tracts contralaterally, which have a high probability of being related to the increased flexor synergy in the patient's left upper extremity. Further, normalizing and maintaining the functional stability of the UGR favorably influences the patient's upright posture and modifies his muscle twitches, which improves his activities of daily living.

Receptor Based Solutions™ for Your Tonic Lumbar Reflex

The Matured Postural Response of the Galant and Modified Galant Reflexes

Introduction

In general, the tonic lumbar reflex is considered to be a more advanced Galant response to gravitational forces. It is an antigravity response of the more evolved or matured nervous system.

Postural Control

The concept of upright posture is achieved by the superposition of body segments along the longitudinal axis. The ability to stand upright has to do with postural components and their primary movers, but there is no universal definition of postural control. There appears to be no agreement regarding the mechanisms that underlie postural and balance functions.

Postural control is a behavior that has to do with the maintenance of body alignment relative to its position in space. That position requires that the body adopt various appropriate upright relationships between various body segments in order to counteract the forces of gravity. This all has to do with the tone of the muscles that would attain and maintain upright posture and vertical stance.

The tonic lumbar reflex is said to be the matured expression of the Galant reflex. Further, the incorporation of the modified Galant reflex lends greater understanding to what it means to stand upright against gravity.

Once stance is achieved, the various body segments—the head, neck, torso, pelvis, extremities—must maintain their center of gravity within specific spatial boundaries related to the individual's base of support. This function requires the ability to maintain equilibrium in space.

Where the Galant reflex provides the ability to facilitate postural patterns, the tonic lumbar reflex is the end result of the mature unification of all the primitive reflex patterns in the lumbar spine.

Posture is primary to the ability to perceive and respond to the environment. It serves to maintain the orientation of the structural segments to their environment, which requires an accurate picture of the position of the body segments with respect to each other and with respect to space. This comes from an accurate postural image that is monitored by multisensory inputs.

There is also a mechanical component to posture. The input from various structural segments must be coupled—or uncoupled—relative to joint stiffness in order to accomplish dynamic tasks.

The tonic lumbar display is an example of the mature coordination of more primitive reflex display. The functional facilitation and inhibition of upper and lower extremities relative to certain laterally deviated body postures helps to maintain appropriate facilitation of spinal cord responses.

The Tonic Lumbar Reflex Display

Certain postural responses to gravitational influences are preprogrammed into the human neurological matrix. The tonic labyrinthine (the reflex that displays a functional facilitation of the flexors in the prone posture and the extensors in the supine posture; a likewise functional inhibition of extensor tone in the prone posture and flexor tone in the supine posture), asymmetric tonic neck, symmetric tonic neck, and Galant reflexes, for example, start as individual primitive reflexes that become assimilated individually and as a group as the human system matures. One example of the functional display of this melding of reflexes is the tonic lumbar reflex.

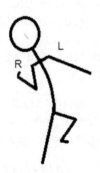

Figure 49: Left convexity/ right concavity

While each of these reflexes are postural, the tonic neck and labyrinthine reflexes appear to have a greater functional influence on the upper extremities than the lower extremities, while the tonic lumbar reflexes and Galant reflexes appear to have a greater functional influence on the lower extremities relative to the upper extremities. Further, any postural reflex may become grossly exaggerated when there is a cortical involvement relative to more neurotypical patients. That is, any deafferentation or hemisphericity can display many of the same findings as a CVA or TBI. This can be demonstrable as a cortical release sign.

The tonic lumbar reflex represents a change in the function of the upper body with respect to the pelvis. The posture will display itself in response to either static upright or dynamic postural changes, or both. The point is that the human neurological fabric will display a response to gravitational influences, but this display may be other than that which is considered appropriate.

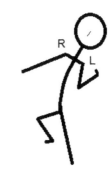

Figure 50: Right convexity/left concavity

In the neurotypical case of right lateral deviation of the lumbar spine on the pelvis (a left convex posture: Figure 49; conversely, right convex posture: Figure 50), the neurological display causes a functional facilitation of the upper extremity flexors ipsilateral to the side of lateral deviation with a concomitant functional facilitation of the lower extremity flexors contralaterally, and a simultaneous functional facilitation of the upper extremity extensors contralaterally and lower extremity extensors, ipsilaterally (Table 11).

Table 11: TONIC LUMBAR REFLEX DISPLAY		
Convexity / Response ↓ →	Functional Facilitation	Functional Inhibition
Left Convexity (Right Concavity)	Right PMC & left latissimus dorsi; Left proximal rectus femoris and distal hamstrings, & right distal rectus femoris	Right latissimus dorsi & left PMC; Left distal rectus femoris & right distal hamstrings
Right Convexity (Left Concavity)	Left PMC & right latissimus dorsi; Right proximal hamstrings, & left distal rectus femoris	Left latissimus dorsi & right PMC; Right distal rectus femoris & left distal hamstrings

The Test Procedure

The tonic lumbar reflex is tested by having the patient lie supine and flat with their hips moved to one side of the table and their shoulders, head, and legs moved to the other side of the table. The patient's posture should be fully convex toward one side with their head laterally bent but kept straight ahead.

The Normal Display

The normal display is a functional facilitation of the upper extremity flexors and lower extremity extensors on the concavity of the curve with a concomitant functional facilitation of the upper extremity extensors and lower extremity flexors on the convexity of the curve. Listen again; there should be a functional facilitation of the clavicular portion of the pectoralis major and gluteus medius, for example, on the concavity of the curve and a functional facilitation of the distal hamstrings on the convexity of the curve. Further, the latissimus dorsi and proximal rectus femoris should be functionally facilitated on the convexity of the curve with a concomitant functional facilitation of the distal rectus femoris on the concavity of the curve.

Summary

The tonic lumbar reflex is essential for afferent reciprocity throughout its homologously related spinal cord segments (Table 12) and it is related to the ability to achieve and maintain upright posture with the concomitant ability to move about within the environment, and it is functionally related and a more mature display of the GR, MGR, and UGR reflexes. All of these reflexes are integral to the various aspects of movement relative to gravity that is so characteristic to the human condition.

Table 12: A COMPARISON BETWEEN THE TONIC NECK AND TONIC LUMBAR REFLEXES		
Body Position (Upright Posture)	Tonic Neck Reflex	Tonic Lumbar Reflex
Stance	Flexion of the head on neck causes facilitation of the upper extremity flexors, bilaterally	Flexion of the head on neck causes facilitation of the upper extremity flexors, bilaterally
Dorsiflexion	Extension of the head on the neck causes facilitation of the upper and lower extremity extensors, bilaterally	Extension of the lumbar spine on the pelvis causes extension of the upper and lower extremity extensors, bilaterally
Ventroflexion	Flexion of the head on the neck causes flexion of the upper and lower extremity flexors, bilaterally	Flexion of the lumbar spine on the pelvis causes flexion of the upper and lower extremity flexors, bilaterally
Rotation	Rotation of the head to the right causes a facilitation of the upper and lower extremity extensors ipsilateral to the side of head rotation and facilitation of the upper and lower extremity flexors, contralaterally	Rotation of the lumbar spine to the right causes facilitation of the upper extremity flexors with a simultaneous extension of the lower extremity extensors ipsilateral to the side of lumbar rotation, and a concomitant facilitation of the upper extremity extensors and lower extremity flexors, contralaterally
Deviation	A right lateral deviation of the head on the neck causes a facilitation of the upper and lower extremity extensors ipsilateral to the side of lateral head deviation and concomitant facilitation of the upper and lower extremity flexors, contralaterally	A right lateral deviation of the lumbar spine on the pelvis causes facilitation of the upper extremity flexors ipsilateral to the side of lateral deviation with a concomitant facilitation of the lower extremity flexors contralaterally, and a simultaneous facilitation of the upper extremity extensors contralaterally and lower extremity extensors, ipsilaterally
Note: A lateral deviation is opposite to the side of convexity; i.e., a right lateral deviation (concavity) is also a left spinal convexity.		

137

Case Study #9

History and Presenting Complaint: Fran; a 28 year old female professional bicyclist. She is in very good athletic shape. She has been working hard with various structural therapies. She recently took a hard fall on a mountain trail and came in to see me with low back pain that radiated through the posterior aspect of her right thigh to her knee.

Examination: The functional neurological examination appeared to show that Fran survived the fall relatively well, but she had some physiological reflex dysfunction that involved her lower back and pelvis. Her patellar and hamstrings deep tendon reflex display appeared to be nominal bilaterally as did her flexor withdrawal, crossed extensor, and Galant reflexes. The piriformis appeared to be functionally inhibited bilaterally without functional facilitation upon ipsilateral head rotation, bilaterally.

The patient was placed supine in the right lateral (a left convex) deviation in order to functionally examine the PMC and hamstrings, bilaterally, with fMMT. The tests revealed a functional inhibition of the PMC and distal hamstrings on the concavity of the lateral deviation, with a concomitant functional facilitation of the PMC and distal hamstrings on the convexity of the lateral deviation.

Imaging: Seven views of the patient's lumbar spine appeared to show a slight reduction of the normal lordotic curve with a dyscoupling bilaterally upon right and left lateral bending, and slight eburnation of the lumbar facets bilaterally more caudally than proximally. The lumbosacral disc space appeared nominal and all other soft tissues appeared to be unremarkable as far as they were visualized.

Clinical Impression: The patient appeared to display an inappropriate functional inhibition of the PMC on the convexity of the lateral deviation and a concomitant functional inhibition of the PMC on the concavity of the lateral deviation—the exact opposite of what one would expect for this functional posture. Further examination indicated a persistent dyscoupling of the third lumbar vertebra that revealed itself secondary to a functionally inhibited piriformis bilaterally, without functional facilitation upon a simultaneous head rotation ipsilaterally. In essence, the patient appeared to sustain a deafferentation of her tonic lumbar reflex with an affiliated reduction in upright stance and postural compromise.

Treatment: The coupled reduction of those lumbar structures demonstrating a resistance to movement enabled the appropriate piriformis display with both ipsilateral and contralateral head rotation. Further, the PMC and hamstrings displayed nominally with both right and left deviation.

Response to Care: The patient was able to immediately arise from the table without her familiar acute pain and her movement was sustained without compromise.

Discussion: The nominal tonic lumbar reflex display supplies its unique symmetrical segmental afferentation to the spinal cord and more rostral neuraxis, which encourages an appropriate motor response to the anterior horn cells of the spinal cord and its segmentally involved muscles. Further, reestablishing the appropriate reciprocal display enables the ability to presynaptically inhibit the nociceptive reflexogenic afferents in the dorsal cord thereby nullifying the nociceptive display and the perception of pain in the patient's right posterior thigh.

Receptor Based Solutions™
for Your Cortical Release Signs

The Modified Galant Reflex Using
Applied Kinesiology as Functional Neurology

Introduction

A number of neurological abnormalities tend to be directly related to the neurological aspects of psychiatric disorders. The prevalence of CRSs in these conditions allows for their use in the clinical management of these patients. However, there are a number of issues that confound the analysis of the CRS's functional display because these dysfunctions are ubiquitous in the general population, they increase in prevalence with age, and there is a lack of specificity and uncertainty over what constitutes an "abnormal" display.

It is clinically important to differentiate a primitive reflex from a CRS. Primitive reflexes are an appropriate infantile display of an inborn neurological response to some external stimulus. An atypical primitive reflex display in the adult is more properly known as a CRS.

The Human Fabric

The Galant Reflex (GR) is an integral part of the normal human neurological fabric at any age. Its pathological display is any functional dysfunction which devolves from that which is unencumbered. This evaluation technique complements the standardized neurological examination and may allow the use of fMMT as an adjunct to the prediction of motor disability in patients of all ages.

Primitive (frontal) reflexes make up some of the earliest, simplest, and most frequently used examination measures to assess the neonate. They are a group of involuntary motor responses normally found early in postnatal development and become intimately and inseparably integrated with the human neurologic fabric. Although their integration is constant, their influence may be "released" by cerebral, usually frontal, damage. (Schott & Rossor, 2003; Hyde *et al*, 2007) Their display becomes pathological when their control mechanisms are mistimed relative to their fundamentals.

Cortical or frontal release signs are common in the general population, occurring in roughly a quarter of young healthy adults, and are more common with advancing age. (Gladstone & Black, 2002) Many researchers have correlated the relationship between primitive reflex display and cognitive impairment. Although a single CRS is of limited clinical significance, multiple CRSs tend to correlate with brain pathology. (Schott & Rossor, 2003) However, the commonly held notion that these reflexes should somehow disappear at certain times has a high probability of being inaccurate. (Walterfang *et al*, 2005)

These reflex patterns are initially distinct and separate at various stages of human development and become integrated into the human neurological fabric consistent with its maturation. The mature neocortex normally keeps higher functional neurological patterns intact. The indications of cortical escape are the motor display of a cortical dysfunction and as such are considered abnormal. Their accumulative effect as a result of a more rostral dysfunction eventually causes a freeing of a group of cortical patterns that later display themselves in the context of CNS disease. The clinical display of these CRSs signifies severe neurological damage when found in the adult, but those same findings may also suggest that they are related to a deafferentation syndrome and can be exposed with MMT. The interpretation of each CRS is described herein with reference to functional neurological norms.

The clinical significance of the demonstrable GR alone, for example, [or in combination with the ATNR, Babinski-like (flexor withdrawal response), and crossed extensor reflexes], as well as their contribution to the early and differential diagnoses of several functional dysfunction syndromes, have been demonstrated in the clinical environment. Moreover, patients with five or more abnormal physiological reflexes have a greater probability of developing associated structural and/or metabolic condition(s). The links between the clinical pictures, CRSs and brain pathology are made clearer with this understanding.

Although a comprehensive neurologic examination is always indicated, the combined examination of primitive reflexes and postural reactions should be considered by the neurologist as a simple but predictive screening test for the early identification of functional neurological issues. A functional neurological examination can elicit many developmental disorders not detected by metabolic screening programs. These neurological screening tests are quick and easy to perform on anyone from neonate to elder adult.

The Muscle-Organ Relationship

Because of its relationship to the homologous intermediolateral cell column, the presence of a functionally dysfunctional GR [together with an aberrant deep tendon reflex (DTR), crossed extensor reflex (CER), or CRS—i.e., tonic neck (TNR), flexor withdrawal (FWR) reflexes] tends to indicate a very high probability that there is a concomitantly dysfunctional autonomic display that involves an associated muscle or muscles.

Further, because of the unique neurological effects of the GR—tapping and stroking the skin in various areas—there appears to be a concomitant display related to the spinocerebellar and the spinothalamic input, respectively. And the outflow from the more rostral neuraxis involves an organic display.

The Cortical Release Signs

By virtue of its homologously-related cord involvement, each of the CRSs has its effect on human movement patterns. They are undeniably involved and inextricably intertwined into the fabric of human movement. These reflexes, when not properly integrated into the maturing CNS, are associated with structural, functional, and autonomic problems. (Guzik *et al*, 2007; Bennett *et al*, 2002)

Joint reciprocity according to the predetermined human design schematic is crucial to functional autonomic display and vice versa. Appropriate and reciprocal joint motion afferentates the spinal cord and more rostral neuraxial centers according to their original intent, and that coordinates appropriate motor responses and autonomic modulation through efferent autonomic drive. This is illustrated in Table 8 above.

The Galant Reflex (GR)

The GR is usually elicited by holding an infant who is prior to its seventh month of age in ventral suspension (face down) and stroking the skin along one side of the lower (below T6) spine. The normal response facilitates the ipsilateral rectus femoris causing the infant to flex at the hip and swing its hips towards the side that was stroked. This normal GR display is raw and unencumbered by other more experienced neurological development. It is said that the GR is pathological if its display persists past six months of age.

Reflexive facilitation of the rectus femoris causes a concomitant inhibition of the ipsilateral hamstring. Therefore, the GR can be used in a clinical setting to evaluate the dynamics of the ipsilateral rectus femoris/hamstring reciprocity (Tables 13 and 14).

Table 13: FUNCTIONAL RECIPROCITY OF THE GALANT REFLEX IN RESPONSE TO STROKING THE LUMBAR FLANK		
Stimulus \ Response ↓ ➝	Ipsilateral Hamstring	Contralateral Hamstring
Stroke Lateral to Lumbar Spine	Inhibition	Facilitation

This paper expands on what has until recently been considered to be the normal GR display for more applicable use in the clinical scenario. This author has observed that stroking and tapping the lateral aspect of the lumbar spine with a sharp object or blunt instrument, respectively, has two different displays. The stroking stimulus causes the ipsilateral rectus femoris' facilitation while the tapping causes its inhibition. Similarly, the crossed cord response causes the opposite display contralaterally. These same stroking and tapping techniques can also be used in the dorsal spine (above T6) with *the opposite* stimulation and display (Table 14).

Table 14: FUNCTIONAL RECIPROCITY OF THE GALANT REFLEX IN RESPONSE TO STROKING OR TAPPING ALONG THE THORACIC AND LUMBAR SPINES		
Stimulation \ Response ↓ →	Ipsilateral Hamstring	Contralateral Hamstring
Stroke Lateral to the Upper Thoracic Spine (Above T6)	Facilitation	Inhibition
Tap Lateral to the Upper Thoracic Spine (Above T6)	Inhibition	Facilitation
Stroke Lateral to Lumbar Spine (Below T6)	Inhibition	Facilitation
Tap Lateral to Lumbar Spine (Below T6)	Facilitation	Inhibition

When the outcome of the fMMT s and their response to the GR tests conforms to their original design, one concludes that its display is nominal. Any other display must be considered pathological.

The GR evaluation consisted of a normal clinical setting. Each patient was tested relative to the GR testing procedures described above. A GR was considered positive when its functional display represented anything other than that which was anticipated by the nominal display. It was difficult to develop a control group because the soft neurological findings appeared ubiquitous. Only after treatment of the patient's individual neurological findings did the dysfunction resolve—become nominal.

Discussion

A number of issues complicate the interpretation of CRSs not the least of which are the myriad observations and interviews reported in the literature. A functional demonstration of the nominal cortical display in the non-clinical population resolves much of the argument. Using fMMT as functional neurology appears to indicate that the understanding of CRSs should be reinterpreted, especially when their clinical significance is persistent and prominent in the examination. In some circumstances, CRSs may assist in diagnostic differentiation and illness staging.

Classical clinical-pathological correlations have suggested that CRSs in adults are one of the few bedside indices of prefrontal cortical dysfunction. (Hyde et al, 2007) If there is a functional display it must have an involved motor component that can be displayed with fMMT.

Conditions of cortical release appear to have a greater neurological consequence relative to normative groups. (Egan *et al*, 2001b; Lawrie *et al*, 2001; Cuesta *et al*, 2002; Gourion *et al*, 2004) However, our data appeared to indicate that dysfunctional CRSs are more common and neurologically involved than previously demonstrated. Those patients who have movement disorders as demonstrated by an aberrant neuromuscular display have learned to utilize some aspect of their primitive reflexes to induce more reliable and predictable movements. This sensory-motor-sensory feedback may show that the persistent yet asymptomatic functional breakdown of the frontal system eventually leads to more profound neurological involvement.

Functional Reciprocity

Functional reciprocity is one of the hallmarks of normal human movement. All primary afferents initially cause excitation to all cord functions including the facilitation of all modulatory effects of the intermediolateral cell column allowing for the dilation of arterioles to muscle and capillaries to skin, and the stimulation of piloerector tissue and sweat glands. They also excite the primary inhibitory neurons that inhibit nociception. Further, their effect rises to midbrain and cerebellar centers. Finally, primary afferents affect all the rostral neuraxial confluence that has any bearing on the anterior horn (the final common pathway), whose effect is reciprocally displayed in each homologously related muscle linked to the initial input.

For the upper and lower extremities to be efficient, besides the shunt stability that makes it possible, the spinal cord signals must maintain reciprocal facilitation of the primary movers and their synergists and inhibition of the ipsilateral antagonists while simultaneously inhibiting and facilitating the muscles that do the opposite activity contralaterally.

Each pre-programmed movement reinforces the interconnectivity between receptors and effectors that maintain the spatial and temporal relationships among the component parts of the movement at the cord levels that share a similar or related structure, position, or function. The synchronicity of the cord with the cortex and midbrain allows for precise and balanced give-and-take motion. With long-term reciprocity, the amount of cortical influence lessens to the point that the component patterns homogenize until a single thought may be sufficient to initiate a whole train of motor events.

Once set, the movement becomes a feedback-regulated pattern that is in some way stored in the CNS fully initiated by a simple but specific input event. The sequence of motor actions can precede almost entirely the control of subcortical means. The functional learning process shifts the major portion of movement control from cortical to peripheral mechanisms.

However, movement patterns tend to degenerate secondary to gravitational influences and their concomitant structural asymmetries resulting in deafferentation of rostral centers and their consequential motor responses. The effect of that deafferentation can be elicited using MMT techniques. Proprioceptive responses can be instantly identified in motor skills inherent to the human genome, and their dysfunction can be quickly diagnosed using functional neurological examination procedures.

A functionally dysfunctional CRS will display itself in a muscle when that muscle is tested with MMT techniques as the result of a timing error—the adjustment of motor planning relative to the sequencing of the muscle function and joint motion such that maximum output power is achieved—somewhere between its receptor, primary afferent, cord involvement, rostral neuraxial centers, cortical outflow, or efferent response. These primitive displays are reflexive, submissive to the primary afferentation that ultimately dictates the integrity of the reflex's display. Other testing procedures monitor the reflexive display but only functional neurological testing observes the efferent response relative to the afferent stimulus. This perspective is the key that distinguishes applied kinesiological procedures as a critical component of functional neurology.

Re-establishing functional central and peripheral reciprocity facilitates cortical integrity and synchrony. Overall, the extensive MMTs helped elicit a physiological display necessary to understand the extent of the dysfunctional CRS's involvement.

Efferent Autonomic Drive and Muscle Concomitants

Only 10% of the entire cortical outflow eventually reaches muscle via corticospinal pathways. Fully 90% of the cortical outflow effects autonomic concomitants via extrapyramidal pathways, and these extrapyramidal pathways modulate the pyramidal display. Of the 10% to muscle, the fibers of the anterior horn must maintain reciprocity lest the dorsal horn of the cord becomes deafferentated, and vice versa.

Each intact CRS has its characteristic display in the human system yet it remains unrecognized unless and until it is challenged. What does it mean to be a "cortical release sign" if that sign is not tested against the function of a muscle? How could a functionally dysfunctional CRS be evaluated other than relative to its functional expression?

Each of these functional displays is important to the mature fabric of the entire human system. Their reciprocal effects influence the cord to allocate movement patterns that respond to the environmental and autonomic factors that support that response. Any influence that generates a dysfunctional motor display will also be accompanied by autonomic concomitants, both of which must ultimately be related to some deafferentation of the higher centers that would create that display, and that ultimately stems from the homologous peripheral receptors.

Further, and because the interdependence of the sensory and motor systems, any individual or combination of dysfunctional CRSs also has its/their negative effect on the integrity of the cortical outflow anywhere from the cortex and rostral mesencephalon to the intermediolateral aspects of the cord. Any deafferentation of the primary afferents—anywhere from the receptor to the cortex—creates a hemisphericity that ultimately displays itself in the performance of a muscle and the function of its related efferent autonomic drive. That outflow is through the extrapyramidal pathways to the cord to segmentally and homologously modulate the involved organs; i.e., organ, vascular, pH, oxygenation, and aerobic performance.

While there may have been an original structural concern, the primary functional lesion may arise from some other homologously-linked area indicating that the original complaint was simply a symptom of a greater picture of abnormal primary afferentation with concomitant dysfunctional efferent autonomic drive. However, when it came to treatment, we considered the global structural involvement and its concomitant autonomic display and not just the focal complaint.

A Receptor-Driven System

The function of the entire human nervous system is receptor-driven. (Godde *et al*, 2003; Weiss *et al*, 2004; Graziano *et al*, 2009; Llinás *et al*, 1999) The whole design is an incredibly dynamic and plastic milieu that is heavily influenced by primary receptor potentiation. Cortical integrity depends on the precision of these primary afferents, which mainly arise from tissues that are able to produce movement of body parts, maintain tension, or pump fluids within the body, influencing even to the most rostral neuraxis.

Nominal cortical efferents cause and modulate both motor and autonomic responses for the benefit of systemic survival giving it insight, texture, and content. The vast majority of this outflow terminates in the areas of the cord that influence functions of the nervous system not under voluntary control, e.g. the regulation of heartbeat or gland secretions, while a relatively smaller percent of these same cortical efferents have their effect on the anterior horn of the cord ultimately exerting their influence on muscle function.

Regardless of their cortical tissue of origin, all the impact from the rostral neuraxis and segmental stimuli finally has its effect on the anterior horn of the cord, the final common pathway. This is where the viscerosomatic system parts ways to affect the muscles and organs according to that specific spinal cord segment, ultimately to cause their own afferent stimuli that finally terminates on the segmental dorsal horn of the cord.

Normalizing Efferent Autonomic Drive

The treatment goal in this procedure was to normalize the dysfunctional efferent autonomic drive secondary to deafferentation of the extrapyramidal and pyramidal outflow that arose as a consequence of a compromised primary afferentation.

Summary

There appears to be uniformity between functional relationships found with the standard CRS's and the results displayed during normal MMT. The demonstrable pathological signs are consistent with a cortical deafferentation and a resultant erroneous motor response. A disruption is demonstrated as any functional display inconsistent with that which was anticipated as normal. These findings strongly indicate that the definition of CRSs should be expanded and used during a standard neurological examination, especially when their clinical significance is sustained and prominent in the examination.

Considering the foregoing, it behooves us to reconsider what it means to have a retained or re-appearing primitive reflex, i.e., reconsider that CRSs are invariably signs of significant brain injury, or at the least a deafferentation of their primary afferent(s). New thought suggests that CRSs are demonstrable in the functional nervous system and any modification of their display indicates a deafferentation of one of the potential neurological levels of dysfunction. The data in this case series suggested that re-establishing functional central and peripheral reciprocity facilitates cortical integrity. The universal goal is to re-establish issues of functional cortical reciprocity in order to achieve purposeful neurological display. Actually, there is much non-drug treatment that can be done for patients with dysfunctional CRS's.

Case Study #10

History and Presenting Complaint: Howard (male, 57yo) sought treatment because of an impending depression the past couple weeks for no apparent reason. He explained that this feeling has been common for him since he was in his early teens. Once it comes on he has a hard time resolving it. He has also had seasonal allergies to pollens, grasses, rye, and animal dander since he was 14 years old. He complains of head congestion and lots of sneezing, enough to be a nuisance at work. He has been taking one Zyrtec per day for the past two to three years.

Examination Findings: During the usual functional neurological examination the patient displayed the following:

Stroking the palm of the patient's hand with a sharp object, bilaterally, appeared to cause the functional inhibition of the clavicular portion of the pectoralis major and hamstrings ipsilaterally with a concomitant functional inhibition of the latissimus dorsi and rectus femoris contralaterally. Stroking the sole of the patient's foot with a sharp object, bilaterally, appeared to cause the functional inhibition of the rectus femoris and latissimus dorsi ipsilaterally with a concomitant functional inhibition of the hamstring and pectoralis major contralaterally.

The Upper Galant reflex in the neutral upright posture: positive bilaterally with both stroking and/or tapping, both above and below T6 when testing the previously functionally facilitated clavicular portion of the pectoralis major and middle deltoid.

The Upper Galant reflex in the seated posture: positive bilaterally with both stroking and/or tapping, both above and below T6 when testing the previously functionally facilitated clavicular portion of the pectoralis major and middle deltoid.

In the seated posture, the bilaterally functionally facilitated rectus femoris and hamstrings remained facilitated when the patient rotated his head ipsilaterally.

In the supine posture, the functionally facilitated left clavicular portion of the pectoralis major remained facilitated when the patient rotated his head ipsilaterally and functionally inhibited when he rotated his head contralaterally.

In the prone position, the Galant reflex appeared to cause the functional inhibition of the previously functionally facilitated hamstrings bilaterally with both stroking and tapping above and below T6, bilaterally.

Imaging: Nine views of the patient's cervical spine were obtained about 18 months previous, which appeared to show a slight right lateral bending of the cervical spine with a concomitant reduction in the cervical lordosis. There appeared to be a dyscoupling of the more distal aspects of the cervical spine with right and left lateral bending. All neuroforaminae appeared to be widely patent bilaterally and all other soft tissues appeared to be unremarkable as far as they were visualized.

(Continued next page)

Case Study #10 *(Continued from previous page)*

Clinical Impression: It seemed reasonable that the dysfunctional flexor withdrawal reflex, Galant display, and concomitant tonic neck reflex display could be the result of a cortical release condition related this patient's depression.

Treatment: The patient received a fast stretch coupled manual manipulative reduction of those structural areas indicating a resistance to stretch. A recheck of the previously dysfunctional findings showed their display to be as anticipated, bilaterally.

Response to Care: The patient responded well to the care given. In his follow up visit he mentioned that his sneezing issues had almost completely resolved and his mood changed significantly after his last visit, and the depression has not returned after three weeks.

Discussion: There were seven functionally dysfunctional primitive reflex indicators positive, and each was positive bilaterally indicating fourteen dysfunctional reflex findings. It is quite possible that the cortical release signs were a consequence of the deafferentation syndrome secondary to the dyscoupled zygapophyseal joint mechanoreceptors of the cervical spine.

Howard's response to reestablishing functional reciprocity through afferent normalization revealed an excellent example of how a dysfunctional afferentation can create a cortical release condition that can display itself without concomitant pain. In this case, the cervical dyscoupling was the efferent response to a functional breakdown of the afferent input.

Over time, the cervical dyscoupling generated dysfunctional primary afferents that produced a deafferentation of the rostral centerline neuraxis with their concomitant display in homologous areas characterized as depression.

Receptor Based Solutions™ for Your Posture

The Human Ability to Stand Upright

Introduction

Posture is simply the position of your body parts assume relative to gravity. It makes no difference whether you are sitting, standing or lying down; your posture displays your body's ability to perform in its environment.

Most people generally assume when we speak of posture it is relative to gravity, but space travelers also have posture where there is no gravity. The absence of gravity makes astronauts assume postures unobserved on earth. For example, their arms rise during sleep or their structure assumes a flexion synergy because there is no stimulation to antigravity muscles.

Good posture is a blessing, but it does not just happen. Standing up straight is not based upon the will to stand upright. Upright posture is a preprogrammed neurological response to gravitational forces. Of course, people can improve their posture when they are reminded to stand up straight or when they realize they are slouching, but without that realization posture is completely unconscious.

The ability to stand, sit or lie down properly has both conscious and unconscious dynamics. Certainly anyone can exhibit any one of the three postures at any given time, but the ability to do it with the proper reflexive responses is one of the keys to good health.

Brief Spinal Observations

The natural, neutral, or healthy spine should be straight when viewed from the back and curved in several places when viewed from the side. (While certain functional issues can be viewed from the front, the spine itself is a posterior structure. Therefore, certain aspects of its functional status can be viewed from the front, for example, in upper and lower limb carriage, hip height, etc.) The spine should have four natural spinal (Figure 51) curves—two lordotic and two kyphotic curves—that sweep forward and backward, respectively. From the top downward, the cervical spine curves forward, the thoracic spine curves backward, the lumbar spine curves forward again and the sacral spine curves backward again. Together, these four curves provide for resilience and the ability to resist

7 Cervical;
Convex forward

12 Thoracic;
Concave backward

5 Lumbar;
Convex forward

5 Sacral

4 coccygeal

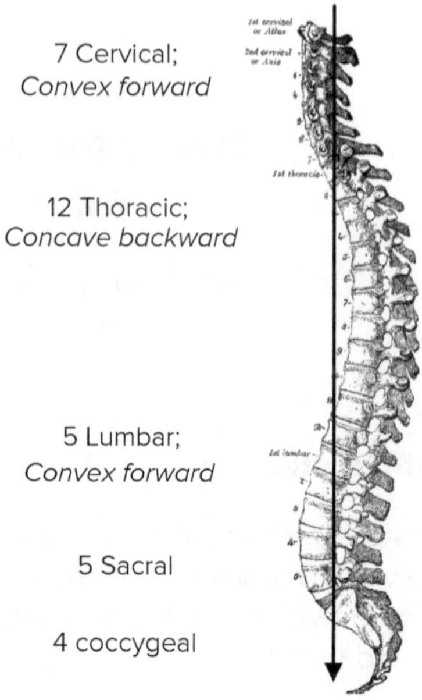

Figure 51: The spine, its vertebra, and various landmarks (Image from Gray's Anatomy 1932)

gravity. This minimizes the stress to the vertebral joints, the core (paraspinal) muscles, and the surrounding tissues.

The fundamentals of upright posture require that a plumb line fall through the anatomical center of the body. From the side view, that line would intersect the back of the ear, through the center of the shoulder joint, through the center of the pelvis, and through the center of the ankles.

From the front view, the plumb line should fall through the center of the head, pass right through the umbilicus, and land equally placed between the feet (Figures 52 and 53).

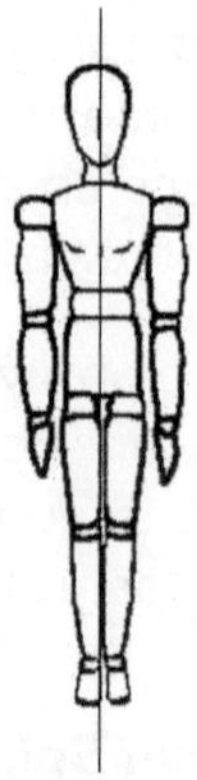

Posture

Of all the characteristics of being human, good posture embodies an effortless bipedal stance—the ability to stand upright against gravity for long periods. But good

Figure 52: Balance: posterior view

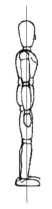

Figure 53: Balance: lateral view

posture does not stop there. We also desire to move around and be productive in our environment. The ability to put one foot in front of the other and move from place to place requires a constant and preprogrammed updating of all the input that would allow that activity. Greater muscle tone produces greater resistance to stretch and faster response to perturbation. The functional spine maintains the optimal alignment of each vertebra to the next while standing, sitting, and/or lying down, with or without movement. The fundamentals of normal human movement support and encourage the proper relationship of spinal mechanics.

In contrast, the dysfunctional spine (Figure 54) is characterized by an inability to function in a productive manner, which leads to an improper gait and stance, especially when walking or standing for long periods. Poor posture puts increased stress on the back that leads to discomfort and structural damage with an increased tendency to injury. Moreover, according to certain laws of orthopedics, bones tend to modify themselves relative to the demands placed on them; a dysfunctional spine modifies or molds itself—the results of polyanionic glycosaminoglycans (PAGs) that create arthritis—as a consequence of postural breakdown. For example, sitting for long periods in ergonomically wrong positions tends to make a person more prone to spinal stress and muscle pain from misalignments and joint breakdown.

The Static Posture

The ability to stand upright stems from many factors, one of which is the positive support phenomenon. It is based on the understanding that putting pressure on the feet as with standing from a seated posture functionally facilitates the muscles that resist gravity. It causes the muscles of the lower extremities to work together to stabilize the body and to support its weight.

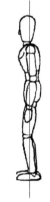

Figure 54: A very poor slouched posture

Watch people as they stand. Check the posture of a friend. See the level of the base of their skull as it sits on the neck. Is it high on one side or low on the other? Next check the evenness of their shoulders. Is one shoulder held higher than the other? Are the shoulder blades level? Does the inside edge of the shoulder blades flare in whole or in part?

Check for any tension in the muscles on one side of the spine relative to the other. The area immediately lateral to the spine is all muscle. Any tension on one side compared to the other can mean that the spinal joints are not moving symmetrically through that area. That can set up hemisphericity that contributes to this structural dysfunction.

Look at the highest part of the hips on each side. Is one hip held higher than the other? Place your thumbs on the hipbone—the posterior superior iliac spine, or PSIS—on either side and ask the patient to slowly lift one knee toward their chest, then the other one. The right response is for the hipbone on the side being tested to rise a bit relative to the hipbone on the other side (i.e., Trendelenburg's test). If the PSIS on the side of the raised leg drops instead of rises, this is an indication of hip joint instability. As a result, you should also check their ankles and feet.

The ankles and feet must bear weight properly; they are the whole body's structural foundation. The feet are the body's first contact with the environment—the earth. No matter what contour the land may be—flat, uneven, soft, hard, etc.—the feet and ankles must respond to it in a functional manner and send their afferents to the cord and brain. As a result, any foot breakdown, such as flat-footedness, for example, can contribute to postural problems and the further breakdown of the antigravity muscles that make the lower extremities take on the form of firm but compliant pillars. Recall what was stated earlier that foot or toe compromise can lead to ankle, knee, and hip involvement.

The Dynamic Posture

In contrast to the static posture, the dynamic posture incorporates the functional movement patterns of the human matrix. A functionally dynamic posture allows and encourages smoothness of gait; it is the embodiment of reciprocity. It moves in predetermined manners that are delightfully human.

An unreciprocated movement pattern is tentative. It is not characterized by a smooth manner and it displays dysfunctional joint stability; it does not allow performance according to the human design.

A Muscle's Optimal Length

In order for a muscle to work optimally it must attain and maintain its optimal length. To pull with purpose the origin and insertion of every muscle must be at their ideal distance apart. Taking that idea a step further, every other muscle must also have its optimal length in order for there to be balance. Their primary afferents create cord symmetry and the efferent response would be equally balanced. But this concept is for discussion only. There is no person alive whose muscles are all at their optimal length; it is a concept, not a reality. Apart from its optimal length—whenever a muscle is in spasm or stretched—its origin and insertion have become too close together or too far apart causing the muscle to become functionally inhibited; it shuts off.

Abnormal Posturing

Poor posture (Figure 54) results when certain muscles tighten up—or shorten (did you know that tight muscles are actually functionally inhibited?)—which weakens them while those muscles that do the opposite function lengthen, functionally inhibiting them, too. This commonly happens when a person's activities of daily living exceed their functional capacity. Their muscles are unable to meet the functional demand being placed on them because their mitochondria (Figure 55) fail to generate the needed ATP, resulting in fatigue in a state of contraction.

Poor posture can show up in several different ways. It can present with rounded and elevated shoulders and/or a forward head placement. This posture places stress on the spine between the top of the neck and skull, and the base of the neck, and upper shoulders. It also leads to shoulder girdle instability, resulting in compromised upper extremity movement patterns. This can also lead to a forward hip tilt, an increased lumbar lordosis with a protruding stomach with stress over both of the hip joints and lower back.

Abnormal posturing is different from "bad posture" or "slouching." An abnormal posture is a deliberate or reflexive tendency to hold a particular body position, or to move one or more parts of the body in a particular way.

Soft and Hard Postural Signs

Normally, when a muscle contracts, the muscles on the opposite side of that joint provide some resistance to contraction to maintain stability. That is a type of posturing—the right type. Certain abnormal postures may indicate specific lesions to the nervous system; these are called hard and soft postural signs. While hard posturing is often observed as an involuntary flexion or extension of the arms and/or legs suggesting severe brain injury, postural abnormalities may also display in more soft functional situations. Abnormal—hard—posturing occurs when frank damage to the CNS (brain and/or spinal cord) results in complete or partial lack of opposition to muscle contraction in various homologously related muscle groups. These hard signs are an important indicator of the amount of brain damage, and are one key to the severity of comatose states in both adults and children.

Other soft postures can indicate some local involvement displaying much the same way as do hard postural signs, but without the frank pathology of tissue damage. Postural signs should always be evaluated by a functional neurologist because many of the soft signs can be returned to normal in order to avoid further structural and functional erosion. The soft postural signs are more often functional, responding to dynamic processing problems in the CNS, but they can often be corrected with certain manipulative therapies. Depending on the state of the nervous system, many hard signs can be made more functional.

The Muscle-Brain-Muscle Link

The functional posture serves as an interface with the external world is actually a group of intermingled reflex responses that maintains body position and equilibrium both during rest—the static posture—and/or during movement—the kinetic posture—by changing the distribution of muscle tone in the head, arm, and trunk. These reflexes can be divided into static and segmental reflexes. The static reflexes maintain equilibrium during rest or non-movement, which include the stretch reflex, the *positive supporting reflex*, and the *negative supporting reflex*. The segmental reflexes involve one or a few spinal segments, such as the stretch reflex, the FWR and the CER.

Of all the characteristics of being human, good posture has to do with the ability to stand upright and move about freely against gravity for long periods. Postural stimulation of the mechanoreceptors from the joints and muscles of the feet contribute to the positive support phenomenon, which converts the lower extremities into well-founded yet conforming columns of support. Merely putting weight on your feet readies a reaction in your spinal cord and brain that enables your whole body to defy gravity with upright posture.

Compression of the foot, as when weight bearing, instinctively evokes facilitation of extensor muscles while traction as in hand suspension facilitates flexors. Similarly, squeezing the bones of the toes together or causing them to be flexed instead of being normally spread apart as if they were jammed into a wrong sized shoe tends to cause all the joints of the lower limb to flex and gravity wins. (This is an excellent reason why shoes must fit right.)

The act of achieving upright posture—putting pressure on the sole of the foot—incorporates a local static stretch reflex from the proprioceptors of the sole of the foot that generates a simultaneous facilitation of the ipsilateral extensor or anti-gravity muscles so that the limb becomes like a rigid support for the body weight. This reflex's center lies in the lumbosacral region of the spinal cord and its display is the positive support phenomenon.

The ability to attain the proper upright posture in any given (earth-bound) environment is the result of the muscle's relationship with the brain, and vice versa. Consider the neurological display of a functionally stable foot. The weight on all its joints is supported by the tone of the muscles and the integrity of their supporting structures, i.e., ligaments, etc. That steady relationship keeps the muscles balanced and the skeleton aligned. Only then can the muscles operate with peak efficiency while reducing the strain on the structure caused by the natural gravitational forces.

Conversely, when the foot's structures become broken down for various reasons, that is, when the foot bones are subluxated, which changes the optimal length of every involved muscle, each episode of weight bearing—every step—generates noxious stimuli to the cord and more rostral neuraxis with a concomitant erroneous motor response to every muscle related to that step.

Similarly, when the pressure is removed from the sole of the foot (as by lifting the lower limb from the floor), relaxation of both extensors and flexors occurs producing a negative supporting reflex. These positive and negative supporting reflexes occur in alternation with each step. These reflexes are also seen in the upper limbs when carrying a heavy object, for example. The center of this reflex lies in the lower cervical and upper thoracic segment of the spinal cord.

Practical Application of Antigravity Technique

The integrity of the positive support phenomenon can be examined by using fMMT (Table 15). Have the patient lie supine and evaluate the middle gluteus medius and hamstrings, bilaterally and note the response. Next, tell the patient to relax their leg and place it into the start position for the medial gluteus medius test. Place the plantar surface of their foot on the middle of your thigh and give a gentle pressure to the patient's straight leg for about 2-3 seconds. Immediately retest that middle gluteus medius. Do the same procedure to the other leg and note the response. Now, bring the patient's legs back to center and give a gentle but firm traction of one to two seconds duration to one of the patient's legs then retest the hamstrings. Do the same to the other leg and note its response. In each case, the muscles tested should be facilitated. This would give you an indication that the patient was responding properly to gravity as far as these tests are concerned.

It is quite possible that the compression to one leg causes the functional inhibition of that middle gluteus medius, indicating the failure of the positive support phenomenon. Further, it is also quite possible that traction to the ipsilateral hamstrings could cause it to become functionally inhibited. Actually, there are several different combinations of positive findings that can result from this series of tests. Keep in mind that the only functionally appropriate response to these tests is the functional facilitation of the muscle being tested and/or the reciprocal functional inhibition secondary to compression or traction.

Muscle \ Action ↓ ➤	Ipsilateral Traction	Contralateral Traction	Ipsilateral Compression	Contralateral Compression
Table 15: ANTIGRAVITY RECIPROCITY TECHNIQUE				
Gluteus medius (Supine)	Inhibited	Facilitation	Facilitated	Inhibition
Hamstrings (Supine)	Facilitated	Inhibition	Inhibited	Facilitation

Antigravity Muscle Function

Antigravity muscles move the bones into their compliant and supporting posture. When these muscles do their job, one could stand forever. However, the truth is that these muscles tend to fail.

How can you tell when the antigravity muscles fail?

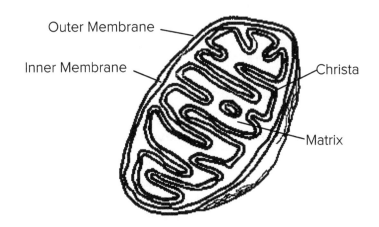

Figure 55: A mitochondria; where ATP is made

Antigravity muscles are designed to contain copious mitochondria (Figure 55), which make ATP to build endurance for upright posture. Muscles need calcium to contract and ATP—from mitochondria—to relax. Therefore, when a muscle fatigues it most often fails in contraction. When the antigravity structure breaks down, the population of these cellular powerhouses wanes and gravity takes over. As a result, muscles that should produce upright posture become feeble leading to joint breakdown and other structural problems.

A misfiring muscle is accompanied by a burning sense in that muscle, which characterizes the presence of too much lactic acid, the result of compromised aerobic metabolism. The joints often ache and movement is often difficult, slowed, and painful. However, there may be no signs or symptoms of muscle problems unless the muscles are functionally tested.

This postural breakdown causes the feet, knees, and hips to flex weakening the lower back. When any one of these three joints of the lower extremity flexes the other two also flex (and, conversely, just for the record, when any one of these three joints extends, the other two also extend). This structural compromise can also affect neck and shoulder posture.

Once the primary afferents reach the cord, interneurons create a broad display that is especially effective in modifying activity in ipsilateral and contralateral muscles, reaching several levels both up and down the cord. Their effects vary with the CIS of the neuronal pool. In other words, if a joint is in flexion it will elicit a different pattern of response than if that same joint is in extension, each condition relative to its homologous involvement.

Testing the Static and Dynamic Postures

Posture is all about the arrangement of the body and its limbs, but it is not a conscious event. Whether good or bad, a person's posture displays the functional nature of their nervous system. It involves the unique way each person carries his or her body as a whole, either intentionally or unintentionally.

An fMMT can reveal the functional nature of these postural supporters. For example, when standing upright in the neutral posture, all antigravity muscles should be functionally facilitated. For example, there are many fMMT's that can be used, but most commonly two basic muscle tests—using the PMC and the latissimus dorsi (LD)—

can give a satisfactory understanding of the function of the upright stance and gait (Table 16).

Once the static posture is examined have the patient step forward comfortable with the right foot, for example, and recheck the PMC and LD for their functional state. Record your findings and have them step back and then forward again with the left foot and again record your findings.

The normal response should be much like the normal gait. When the right foot steps forward the normal gait response is for the left upper extremity to also swing forward. In essence, this is because the muscles of the right upper hip have functionally facilitated with a consequential functional inhibition of the muscles that would have otherwise caused extension of that leg and a simultaneous functional facilitation of the ipsilateral upper extremity extensors and functional inhibition of the ipsilateral upper extremity flexors. Contralaterally, with the forward swing of the left upper extremity comes an associated functional facilitation of the flexors of that extremity and a concomitant functional inhibition of the ipsilateral upper extremity extensors. Finally, the left lower extremity follows the same scheme, reciprocally. That is, the functional facilitation of the lower extremity extensors and a functional inhibition of the ipsilateral lower extremity flexors.

Table 16: NORMAL DISPLAY OF UPRIGHT STANCE AND GAIT USING THE PMC AND LD			
Muscle \ Stance or Gait → ↓	Neutral	Right Foot Forward (RFF)	Left Foot Forward (LFF)
Ipsilateral PMC	Facilitated	Inhibited	Inhibited
Contralateral PMC	Facilitated	Facilitated	Facilitated
Ipsilateral LD	Facilitated	Facilitated	Facilitated
Contralateral LD	Facilitated	Inhibited	Inhibited
PMC: Clavicular division of the Pectoralis Major; LD: Latissimus Dorsi			

Functional Manual Muscle Tests (fMMT) for Stance and Gait

The Test: With the patient standing in their natural and neutral upright stance with their head straight ahead and their eyes open, test the PMC and LD bilaterally and make a note of any patterns of functional facilitation and/or functional inhibition.

Next, have the patient take a comfortable step forward with either foot and be sure their head is straight ahead during the test. The step must be natural and the patient must have their weight on their front foot with the ball of their back foot staying in contact with the ground. Test the PMC and LD again and note any patterns of functional facilitation and/or functional inhibition.

Finally, have the patient step back to their neutral stance and then step forward again with the other foot. Be sure that the step is natural, that their head is straight ahead, and that the patient has their weight on their front foot with the ball of their other foot in contact with the ground. Test the PMC and LD again and note any patterns of functional facilitation and/or functional inhibition.

Normal Response: The natural display in the neutral stance is a functional facilitation of each PMC and LD, bilaterally.

When the patient strikes a gait posture with either foot, it is normal for the contralateral PMC and ipsilateral LD to be functionally facilitated and for the ipsilateral PMC and contralateral LD to be functionally inhibited. Consider each of these postures relative to the walking gait. When a foot comes forward the opposite arm also swings forward. What are the muscles that move these extremities into these postures? Those are the muscles that should be facilitated and the antagonists should be inhibited.

Pathological Response: Any display other than the normal response above should be considered to be pathological. That is, there may be a functional facilitation of all muscles, a functional inhibition of all muscles, or any combination of functional facilitation and/or functional inhibition of all muscles other than that which is normal, and each of these presentations should be considered pathological.

Summary

Posture is that structural and autonomic expression that allows humans to maintain a functional and bipedal ability within their environment. Upright posture is one of several uniquely human traits. It only makes sense that that movement should be symmetrical and reciprocal, and accompanied by balance. Every movement requires balance and stability, and an associated autonomic concomitant to nourish the muscles that are under functional demand. However, as a result of inappropriate sensory input, the functional posture can easily lose its stability, and that is when joint and muscle problems develop leading to various types of aches and pains, and an increased potential for injury. Structural compromise also involves organ function, especially the eyes and ears, and the ability to remain upright in one's own environment. Therefore, it is essential for the doctor to know how to understand each postural display and resolve it to the best of their—and the patient's—ability.

Case Study #11

History and Presenting Complaint: Ralph (85 year old male) presented with acute discomfort in his lower back and left cervicodorsal spine. He enjoys working out with light weights every morning, but there was no specific traumatic event related to his discomfort. The patient has a history of making several hundred parachute jumps while in the military.

Exam Findings: fMMT of the gluteus medius and hamstrings in the supine posture displayed a normal functional facilitation. There appeared to be an associated functional facilitation of the gluteus medius on the right upon simultaneous compression of the ipsilateral lower extremity, but a functional inhibition of the gluteus medius on the left after a similar test. The right hamstrings appeared to be functionally facilitated immediately after traction of that lower extremity and a functional inhibition of the left hamstring after a similar test ipsilaterally.

The clavicular portion of the pectoralis major (PMC) and the middle deltoid (mDelt) muscles appeared to be functionally nominal bilaterally in the upright and supine postures. However, when in the seated posture, the PMC and mDelt were unable to meet the demands of manual muscle testing. Further evaluation indicated functional facilitation of both the PMC and mDelt upon challenging the L5 in a +theta Y direction.

Imaging: Seven views of the lumbar spine revealed a loss of the normal lordosis with an abnormal coupling upon right and left lateral bending of his lumbar spine. All views appeared to show a chronic DJD, with a associated reduction in the joint space between L4/5 and L5/S1. The neuroforamina all appeared to have lost a good degree of patency and there appeared to be significant eburnation of the lumbar facets bilaterally and throughout. All other soft tissues appear to be unremarkable as far as they were visualized.

Clinical Impression: The normal movement patterns of the lower back appear to have been compromised contributing to this patient's lower back pain.

Treatment: The patient was placed in the right decubital posture and L5 was manipulated with a coupled manual technique.

Response to Care: When the PMC, mDelt, gluteus medius and hamstrings were retested, each appeared to function nominally, bilaterally.

Discussion: The foregoing case is an excellent example of the functional effect of a dysfunctional positive support phenomenon. The left lower extremity was unable to properly respond to postural stimulation with a concomitant inhibition of those left lower extremity muscles that should have otherwise been able to withstand the demands being placed on them. Further, the functional compromise of the lower body had its concomitant effect in the upper extremity of the same side.

Postural stability is essential for meaningful human abilities. Any structural breakdown has its functional display.

Section III

Receptor Based Solutions™ for Your Application

Rats in Space

The Neurology of Spinal Erection

Introduction

The entire experience of human existence is based upon the gravitational effects of joint mechanoreceptor stimulation secondary to joint movement, and joint movement is a result of muscle function. The ability to resist the Earth's gravitational field is the result of postural muscles, through cerebellar reflex pathways. No function of human existence in our Earth-bound existence is independent of gravitational forces and their effect upon joint mechanoreceptor potentiation.

During the first part of November 1993, the Orange County Register ran a story entitled, "Space Rats Shed Light on Muscle Mechanics." This story took place at about 250 miles above the earth in the Space Shuttle, Columbia. Researchers at the University of California at Irvine closely monitored five rats that spent two weeks in low earth orbit. The scientists wanted to understand more about the results of short duration space flight on endurance muscle function. The researchers said their findings might mean an end to the idea that we are made of just two types of muscle—one for endurance activities and one for quick bursts of activity.

Once the rats safely returned to earth, they were sacrificed and dissected, and their muscles were studied closely. The results of the studies showed that the rats lost 30 percent of their endurance muscle function during the flight.

The researchers found it interesting that the rats lost mostly slow-twitch (or type I) muscle—that type of muscle used for endurance activity such as distance running—and relatively little fast-twitch (type II) muscle—that muscle tissue used for short bursts of activity such as sprinting.

Further, they were also surprised to find that some, but not all of the slow-twitch muscle fibers began to adapt into fast-twitch muscle fibers during the flight. One of the researchers was quoted as saying, "We need to explore further why some can change and the others cannot." Characterizing how muscle loss occurs is the first step toward understanding how to treat it, they said. The understanding of this type of change can benefit not only astronauts, but also the infirm and elderly, who often suffer tremendous muscle loss."

Another researcher said, "We need to learn a lot more about how we can offset these changes, but first we need to know the types of changes that are occurring."

Discussion

Types of Muscle

Muscles are generally distinguished histochemically into two basic types. One type corresponds to the fast-twitch (type II) fibers; the predominant metabolic enzymes present in these muscle fibers are related to anaerobic (glycolytic) metabolism. The other type relates to the red slow-twitch (type I) fibers, which rely primarily on oxidative metabolism.

Ability to Make ATP

Besides being defined as fast and slow twitch fibers, muscles can also be categorized by their ability to resist fatigue. Slow twitch muscles are aerobic and possess a high degree of endurance character. They function to resist gravity; they are generally extensor or postural (shunt) muscles. They contain more mitochondria and therefore more mitochondrial electron acceptors (MEA's), more sarcoplasmic reticulum and a higher population of contractile proteins. Aerobic muscles also have a greater ability to produce ATP and replicate protein than that of anaerobic muscles. As a consequence of a decreased level of joint mechanoreceptor stimulation, aerobic muscles adapt to become more like anaerobic muscles. They lose their mitochondrial electron acceptors, they contain less sarcoplasmic volume, and they have a diminished ability to aerobically produce ATP and replicate proteins at a high rate.

The ATP necessary for aerobic muscle function is generally produced via the Krebs Citric Acid Cycle, which is readily found in the mitochondria of type I muscles. When the essential components for the successful completion of the citric acid cycle are available, there are about 36 molecules of ATP produced. However, if this cycle cannot be completed because of the unavailability of the requisite factors, not only does the total number of ATP molecules drop from 36 to 2, but also the ATP production must be shifted to anaerobic (the Emden-Myeroff, for example) pathways leading to an overall decrease in the production of energy. Not only do the anaerobic pathways yield fewer molecules of ATP, but they also lead to an increased production of lactic acid, which is a well-known tissue irritant.

Under normal circumstances, during muscular exercise, the muscle's blood vessels dilate and blood flow increases to enhance available oxygen supplies. Up to a point, the increase in oxygen consumption is proportionate to the energy expended, and aerobic processes meet all the energy needs. However, when muscular demands exceed the autonomic capacity to meet these demands, aerobic processes fail. This is when phosphocreatine is used to resynthesize ATP.

Phosphocreatine resynthesis is accomplished by using the energy released by the anaerobic breakdown of glucose to lactic acid. This use of the anaerobic pathway is self-limiting, because in spite of the rapid diffusion of lactic acid into the blood stream, enough lactic acid accumulates in the muscles to eventually exceed the capacity of the tissue buffers and produces an enzyme-inhibiting decline in the muscle tissue's pH. However, for short periods, the presence of an anaerobic pathway for glucose breakdown permits muscular exertion of a far greater magnitude than would be possible without it. Without this anaerobic pathway, for example, walking or running at a slow jog would be possible, but it would be impossible to sprint or do other forms of quick exertion.

Cerebellar Stimulation

The cerebellum innervates paraspinal muscles through subconscious means. The cerebellum receives its stimulation almost completely through the afferentation from large diameter—type Ia—axons that arise from muscle spindles, and type I and II joint mechanoreceptors.

These receptors are organized with a higher population and priority, oriented more rostrally than caudally. Therefore, these receptors are more sensitive to spinal, costosternal, costotransverse, and costovertebral articular motion than other types of joint activity. Their axons rise to the level of the cerebellum mainly through spinocerebellar and cuneocerebellar pathways, and terminate in midline cerebellar centers (Figure 56). From here, efferent axons travel via the fastigiovestibular tract to all four vestibular nuclei in the area acoustica in the floor of the fourth ventricle (Figure 57). These nuclei send fibers both rostrally and caudally to coordinate higher centers with joint motion (Figure 58). The caudal-projecting fibers make up the vestibulospinal tracts, both medial and lateral. These nuclei are at their CIS because of cerebellar afferentation and cause paraspinal muscle stimulation, and therefore spinal extension and upright posture.

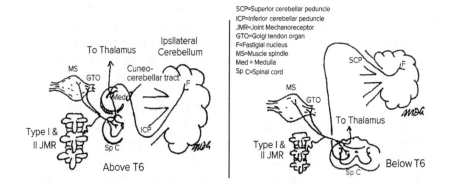

Figure 56: Cerebellar afferents

Spinal Joint Motion

There is no conscious way to move one vertebra relative to another. Each of the paraspinal muscles is subconsciously innervated via the cerebellum and vestibular nuclei. The rostral-projecting fibers arise from the superior, medial, and inferior vestibular nuclei, to make up the medial lemniscus and terminate in the Oculomotor (III), Trochlear (IV) and Abducens (VI) nuclei to coordinate extraocular movements with spinal function; ocular and spinal movements are said to be hard-wired.

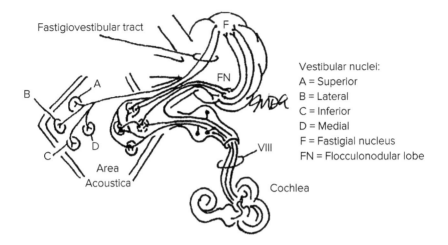

Fastigiovestibular tract

Vestibular nuclei:
A = Superior
B = Lateral
C = Inferior
D = Medial
F = Fastigial nucleus
FN = Flocculonodular lobe

Area Acoustica

Cochlea

Figure 57: Cerebellar efferents to the vestibular nuclei

Cerebellar Drive

The cerebellum drives the mesencephalic and thalamic centers, particularly the red nucleus and reticular formation through the decussating dentatorubroreticulothalamic tract, and from there to all cortical centers through the corona radiata (Figure 59). These centers, together with those fibers from the thalamus, drive the extrapyramidal cascade (Figure 60) via the thalamohypothalamoreticulospinal pathway, which synapses in the brainstem to drive cranial nuclei III, VII, IX and X, the pontine and medullary reticular formations through the fastigioreticular tract (Figure 61), as well as the medullary respiratory and many other centers.

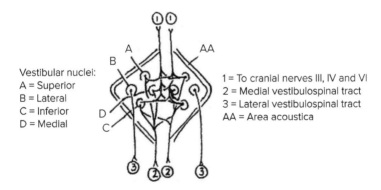

Vestibular nuclei:
A = Superior
B = Lateral
C = Inferior
D = Medial

1 = To cranial nerves III, IV and VI
2 = Medial vestibulospinal tract
3 = Lateral vestibulospinal tract
AA = Area acoustica

Figure 58: Vestibular efferents

Review of the Foregoing

As a result of spinal and rib mechanics, the receptor potential from the zygapophyseal mechanoreceptors of the centerline skeleton causes stimulation of more rostral centers, which return motor response to all the areas they innervate and cause a neurophysiological reaction based upon that receptor input. Therefore, it is reasonable to say that the process of respiration is dependent upon mechanoreceptor afferentation. Without mechanoreceptor afferentation, respiratory centers would be dysfunctional; and that is exactly what happens!

Extrapyramidal Outflow

Going one step further, the thalamohypothalamoreticulospinal tract exerts an inhibitory effect upon the anterior muscles above T6 and the posterior muscles below T6. This provides a modulation of the strong facilitory effect to these same muscles produced via the corticospinal outflow from contralateral centers.

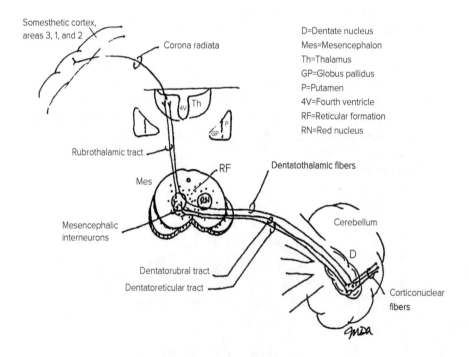

Figure 59: Cerebellar efferents to the cortex

Generally, a muscle will continue to perform according to its metabolic abilities unless and until these needs change due to a change in metabolic demand—i.e., the muscle undergoes modified G-forces, the joint sustains a subluxation, it experiences disuse, overuse, or overtraining, it suffers some other degenerative changes, or the essential components for repair are no longer available, etc. Moreover, a muscle will only produce contractile proteins relative to their need.

In a zero-G environment, there is a decreased need for any type of muscle function, especially for those of the antigravity type. Therefore, any change in demand that modifies the spinal extensor muscle's ability to function normally causes the juxtaposed muscle(s) to undergo disuse atrophic changes. The endurance muscle adapts from the type I muscle and takes on an appearance much the same as that of a type II muscle. That is, the muscles are less able to sustain endurance (shunt) activity and more willing to perform short burst (spurt) endeavors; they change from an aerobic to an anaerobic type. This is accompanied by an inability to function as originally designed, and that leads to:

- Neuropathophysiology: global deafferentation; immune and inflammatory responses;
- Myopathology: muscle atrophy;
- Histopathology: connective tissue and vascular pathology;
- Kinesiopathology: pathological changes in muscle function;
- Biochemopathology: deficiency of the essential components for repair;
- Bioelectropathology: inability to propagate an adequate neurophysiological impulse

Shunt and Spurt Characteristics

When discussing fast and slow twitch muscles, it is important to also discuss shunt and spurt characteristics of those muscles. Each has a particular function related to joint stabilization. Shunt muscles are those muscles that provide joint stability. By definition, a shunt muscle is one whose origin is closer to the joint than its insertion, giving it a greater ability to stabilize a joint (Figure 62). A spurt muscle, on the other hand, is a joint mover. Its origin is further away from the joint than its insertion; it acts as a lever.

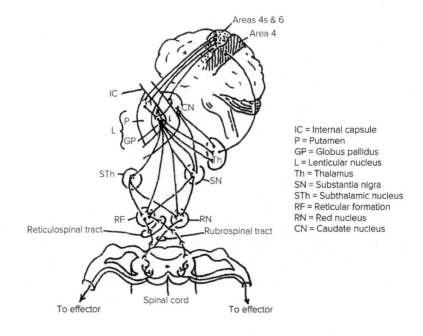

IC = Internal capsule
P = Putamen
GP = Globus pallidus
L = Lenticular nucleus
Th = Thalamus
SN = Substantia nigra
STh = Subthalamic nucleus
RF = Reticular formation
RN = Red nucleus
CN = Caudate nucleus

Figure 60: Extrapyramidal pathways

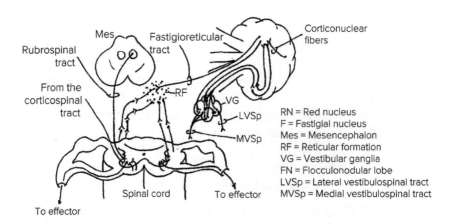

RN = Red nucleus
F = Fastigial nucleus
Mes = Mesencephalon
RF = Reticular formation
VG = Vestibular ganglia
FN = Flocculonodular lobe
LVSp = Lateral vestibulospinal tract
MVSp = Medial vestibulospinal tract

Figure 61: Cerebellar efferents to the cord

It is possible for a muscle to act as a shunt muscle in one activity and as a spurt muscle in another activity. An example of this is the stability produced between the spine and scapula in order for the first 90 degrees of upper extremity abduction to occur. In this instance, the spine and scapula are stabilized by shunt muscles and provide the steadiness necessary for spurt muscles to produce the activity of upper extremity motion. In the second 90 degrees of upper extremity abduction, the spinal shunt muscles act individually to provide stabilization of the vertebrae while those muscles that previously provided scapular shunt stability now function differently to provide the spurt activity of scapular rotation and upper extremity movement.

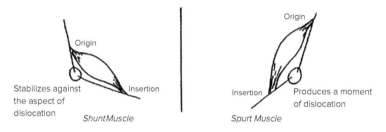

Figure 62: Shunt and spurt muscles

The Effect of Atrophic Change

As muscles atrophy, shunt muscles lose their aerobic ability to stabilize a joint; they lose their capacity to endure and the involved joint becomes unstable. When spurt activity is superimposed upon an unstable joint, it causes the breakdown of the polyanionic glycosaminoglycans of joint cartilage, leading to degenerative joint disease and further deafferentation of that joint. Moreover, an atrophied muscle's endurance activity wanes in favor of a short burst modification, resulting in a change from aerobic to anaerobic metabolism. If this metabolic breakdown happens in the vertebral zygapophyseal joints, there is a very high probability that the cerebellum and dentatorubroreticulothalamic tracts would become deafferentated, as would those higher centers of the mesencephalon and thalamus with a consequentially negative modification of the modulatory effects of the thalamohypothalamoreticulospinal tract, leading to a concomitant decrease in the CIS of the autonomic and ocular-related cranial nerves III, IV, VI, VII, IX and X, and oxygen utilization, as well as bringing about a change in pH to a more acidic level as related to a drive toward potassium equilibrium potential in these areas.

Further, since the thalamohypothalamoreticulospinal tract acts to inhibit the ipsilateral anterior muscles above T6 and the ipsilateral posterior below T6, the hyperpolarization of this inhibitory tract via the deafferentation of its afferents ultimately causes a facilitation of that postural function, and the trunk and extremities do that which they are normally inhibited from doing. That is, the ipsilateral upper extremity flexors and lower extremity extensors become facilitated, creating the neurologic equivalent of a stroke antalgia.

Changes in Optimal Pull

A change in muscle contractibility also alters its length. When a muscle loses its optimal length, that is, when a muscle's origin and insertion become either too close together or too far apart, which can happen as a result of a subluxation or a zero-G environment for example, the muscle length changes and its ability to perform useful work decreases.

In a zero-G environment, postural muscles are unnecessary and they produce less ATP. Actually, ATP is not needed for muscles to contract; it is only needed to release a contraction. To change atrophied slow twitch muscle fibers back to normal slow twitch fibers, its mitochondrial substrate, and sarcoplasmic volume must be enhanced. In order for a muscle to become stronger, it requires tetany in that muscle, which leads to increased protein replication.

Functional Zygapophyseal Rehabilitation

Rehabilitation of spinal joints requires cerebellar depolarization through stimulation of type Ib afferents via fast stretch coupled manual manipulation to the structures demonstrating a resistance to motion, and resultant stimulation to the types I and II joint mechanoreceptors. This stimulates cerebellar function and a drive toward sodium equilibrium potential and a resultant increase in the CIS of the vestibular nuclei, with consequential increase in supraspinal control over the paraspinal musculature. The more stimulation these muscles receive, the more work they can do. The more muscle strength created, the more tension can be produced, and the more binding sights can be developed. This leads to an enhanced joint juxtaposition and greater functional stability, and an enriched central integration of this afferentation.

Human Need for Gravity

If a vertebra is truly misaligned or subluxated, so that the amplitude of receptor potentials in that joint is decreased as a component of reduced mechanical stress, then the detrimental effects of gravitational loading on the joint is a concern. That makes this "Rats in Space" model very appropriate and only reinforces our dependence on Earth and our inborn ability—and necessity—to correctly resist gravity's attraction. The ability to withstand gravity is via the utilization of the central integration of afferentation as a consequence of the gravitational pull; i.e., all other influences being intact, the ability to stand erect is directly proportional to the amount of joint mechanoreceptor stimulation generated as a consequence of stretch.

With the foregoing in mind, consider that it only takes six to ten days for a muscle to lose half of its ability to perform useful work. In the next six to ten days, half of what is left is lost and so forth until after 30 days, up to 90 percent of a muscle's functional capacity can be lost. This relates equally to a spinal subluxation and to a zero-G environment. The longer each exists, the more problems they produce and the longer it takes to fix them, if at all. The rehabilitation of an atrophic muscle is possible if no joint degenerative changes have occurred. However, if degeneration has begun, full rehabilitation is less likely due to the resultant structural and functional deafferentation of the joint.

Summary

The "Space in Rats" experiment revealed a 30 percent adaptation in endurance muscle function after just two weeks. In humans, we know this number to be approximately 50 percent in just six to ten days. One main obvious difference is that humans are bipeds—one of many uniquely human characteristics—while rats are quadrupeds; a human's cerebellar connectivity is vastly more developed than that of a rat. Therefore, the functional consequences of both the ability to maintain upright posture and the dysfunctional effects of metabolic breakdown in human neurology is much more complicated than any other animal.

The last sentence of the last paragraph of the newspaper article reads, "We need to learn a lot more about how we can offset these changes, but first we need to know the types of changes that are occurring."

Let me tell a story that will help make the point. There is a man who runs in my neighborhood. I see him every day. His workout is so regular you could set your clock by him. His run is not very fast but it is peculiar. His elbows are flexed and they never reach behind his midline. His knees are quite flexed and he runs on his toes. His feet never go very far backward. As I watch him run I realize that his posture is rather flexed. His metabolism is so anaerobic—overtrained—that his spinal shunt stabilizers are in spasm and his posture is actually in extension. He has to run with such a flexed posture to overcome his posteriorly displaced center of pressure. His spinal muscles are so compromised from type I fibers to type II fibers that if he ran more upright he might fall backward!

When you consider the impact of Orange County Register's Space Rats article, it is sad that with all the spinal dysfunction—subluxations—out there, that we have to send billion dollar mice up into space to discover what the chiropractic profession has clinically realized for over a hundred years and functional neurology can easily explain.

The first step of spinal rehabilitation is to reestablish functional joint position sense in the shunt muscles by working axially and moving peripherally. Only then can attention can be paid to the spurt muscles. It is imperative to reestablish the metabolic function of the shunt muscles that have adapted to become spurt-like. If shunt stability is forgotten then the structural problems will persist with continued neuropathophysiologic, myopathologic, histopathologic, kinesiopathologic, biochemopathologic, and bioelectropathologic breakdown. Adapted shunt muscles must regain the stabilizing function they once provided; i.e., the ability to use oxygen, increase their number of mitochondria and mitochondrial electron acceptors, expand their ability to replicate proteins at a high rate, and to boost their sarcoplasmic reticulum.

The researchers in the article were looking at the zero-G environment of low earth orbit and appeared to be asking the question, "Why did we see type I muscle fibers change to look like type II fibers, but the type II fibers did not change to look like type I fibers?" There are so many variables and it is more than the result of zero-G. Many neurological components must be added to the equation and without them; this question is actually one of futility.

Chiropractic has innately recognized the importance of proper spinal function for over a century. Our philosophy has been cramped not as a consequence of its inadequacies, but as a consequence of the inadequacies of science and technology heretofore. A medical researcher might look at this study and ask, "Why?" The chiropractic neurologist might look at the exact same research and say, "Why not?"

Chiropractic is not medicine and refuses comparison. Any link tends to make chiropractic doctors sound like they want to be like medical doctors. However, the comparison of their fundamental differences is futile. The basic medical model of comparing two variables and drawing conclusions is not appropriate for the interpolation of the wonders of specific modulation and the evocation of those things that are always changing.

Surround Inhibition

Discussion of the Miracle of Upright Posture

Introduction

The human body is made up many different systems – circulatory, respiratory, immune, musculoskeletal, excretory, genitourinary, endocrine, digestive and nervous. Each system has its own purpose and is functionally dependent upon all the others in order to work properly. The first of the organized fetal systems to work as a functional unit is the nervous system, first making its appearance about 21 days after conception; before most women know they are even pregnant (Table 17).

In just over 500 hours, a fertilized egg differentiates into a neural tube and then into three parts: the prosencephalon (forebrain), the mesencephalon (midbrain) and the rhombencephalon (hindbrain). The prosencephalon divides into the telencephalon and diencephalon. The mesencephalon remains undifferentiated throughout its existence. The rhombencephalon divides into the metencephalon and the myelencephalon. From these primitive parts come all the other components of the human nervous system. Our discussion regarding surround inhibition, however, will remain confined, for the most part, to the area of the rhombencephalon—that area containing the cerebellum and pons (both from metencephalon)—and the other nuclei and tracts (myelencephalon) of particular interest to our subject.

Starting from the first manifestation of the human nervous system, this chapter will describe a novel functional interpretation of surround inhibition (Figure 66) that may help clarify the role of the cerebellum in movement control. Briefly, the cerebellum is a functional grid of "beams" that receive certain sequences of input and responds in signals of output. These functional events are typical of the cerebellar cortex. Purkinje cells respond to sequences of stimuli in the mossy fiber system as a result of movement display. The sequences of mossy fiber activation that normally produce this effect in the intact cerebellum are a combination of motor planning relayed to the cerebellum by the cerebral cortex, and information about ongoing movement that reaches the cerebellum from the spinal cord. The output elicited by the specific sequence to which a "beam" is tuned may well be a succession of well-timed inhibitory volleys "sculpting" the motor sequences so as to adapt them to the complicated requirements of the physics of a multi-jointed system.

Table 17: DIFFERENTIATION OF EMBRYONIC TISSUES

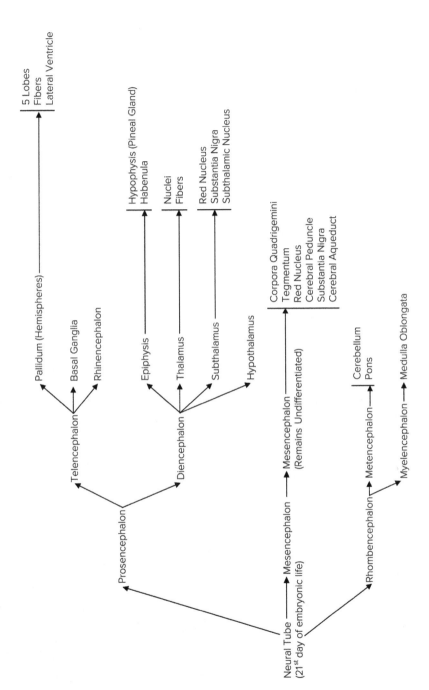

Our primary focus here is on the cerebellum and its homologous structures. As is true with the whole human neuraxis, none of its parts can function without some way of telling what is happening in the body as a whole, and to relate each of these areas to the others. The cerebellum is uniquely qualified to do that specific job. It relates to each of the body's systems and orchestrates their synchrony (Figure 63).Of all the parts of the nervous system, and relative to the other aspects of human brain function, the tasks of the cerebellum are some of the least understood and discussed. Yet, the cerebellum's part in the performance of the entire nervous system is vital in examining and responding to the incoming neuromuscular input from every area of the neuraxis.

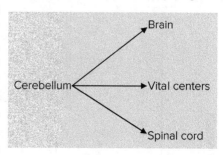

Figure 63: Cerebellar connections

The input to the cerebellum comes from various places and is assimilated for use in comparison to all other areas of input. The information is then distributed to the motor and autonomic pathways for response and awaits the receipt of new and updated information.

The cerebellum ("little brain") lies inferior to the cerebral hemispheres and posterior to the upper brainstem structures of pons and midbrain. The visible portion of the cerebellum is a thin layer of highly corrugated (grooved) gray matter—the cerebellar cortex. The core of the cerebellum contains the white matter. The cerebellum may be broadly divided into the midline structure called the vermis ("worm") and two lateral cerebellar hemispheres (Figure 69).

The cerebellum is the chief brain structure for coordination of muscle groups (synergy), regulation of muscle tone and degree of muscular contraction, and performance of rapid, precise, coordinated movement patterns. The cerebellum largely determines the speed, range, and synchronization of movements. Primarily, it fills in the bumps and snarls of incoming signals and smoothes out the response to them. It coordinates movement, compares intended and actual movement and corrects for differences, is involved in motor learning, has an output to the premotor and motor cortex through the thalamus, and has an output to the brainstem.

One of the most important secrets about the cerebellum is that it receives no input arising from the osseous portion of joints. The sole cerebellar input from the structure comes from the large diameter afferents from muscle spindles and Golgi

> The cerebellum's chief concern is to synchronize the actions of the various body systems.

tendon organs, and the surrounding soft tissues. The input from these same structures, including their bony input and that input from all other areas—except that of smell—must go through the thalamus before reaching the cerebral cortex.

The motor control hierarchy proceeds from the motor cortex to the brain stem and spinal cord. The cerebellum and basal ganglia are also intricately involved to provide modulatory loops that are important for proper motor control.

Cerebellar lesions produce ipsilateral effects because the output pathways from the cerebellum decussate and integrate with pathways that again cross over to the side of the original cerebellar output. Symptoms of damage to the cerebellum include hypotonia (poverty of movements), asthenia (tiring of muscles), decomposition of movement (puppet-like movement), dysmetria (an inability to estimate distance accurately), dysdiadochokinesia (inability to perform rapid repetitive and alternating movements of which oral dysdiadochokinesis is a special case), ataxic gait (awkward, staggering movements) and intention tremor (fine shaking upon voluntary movement). Cerebellar lesions cause dysarthria (imperfect articulation of speech due to disturbances of muscular control).

The rest of this chapter discusses cerebellar anatomy, afferents, efferents, vascular control, modulation of vital centers, cerebellar lesions and treatment application to help people reach the level of health they desire; to help sick people get well and keep well people from getting sick.

Part 1: Cerebellar Anatomy

The cerebellum's chief concern is to synchronize the actions of the various body systems. Each system must know what the other systems are doing, and none is isolated from the others. When the signals from the different aspects of human function are combined with the help of cerebellar analysis, the systemic effect is greater than would be expected from any of the different aspects acting separately. For example, the initiation or perpetuation of movement requires the contraction of a muscle or a group of muscles. At the same time, however, those muscles that oppose that initial action must relax. Also, movement requires a specific quantity of muscle contraction. The amount of contraction can only be adjusted by the number of muscle fibers involved in the reaction, which, in turn, is a function of the number of nerve fibers activated. Further, movement requires the proper duration of the nerve impulses for the completion of an act. Finally, when movement requires motion at several joints, it is essential for muscles to contract and relax in proper sequence.

The sum total of all cerebellar afferents requires a competent response that coordinates the synergy of purposeful movement. Therefore, the cerebellum has earned the nickname as an "error comparer" because it is involved in every aspect of the humanity.

In order for all these intricacies of motion to occur, certain basic connections must be present (Figure 64). First, the cerebellum must receive a continuous inflow of adequate information from the muscular system regarding the state of muscle tension. Constant streams of input data set up by movements must reach the cerebellum form the soft tissues of the joints. Another type of input must reach the cerebellum from the vestibular receptors in the inner ear. At the same time, the cerebellum must be intimately linked to the streams of impulses leaving the voluntary motor centers of the cerebrum. While all this is going on, the cerebellum must contain an internal organization which will coordinate this information and it must possess properly organized efferent pathways so that it can exert its influence upon the segmental apparatus and lower motor centers.

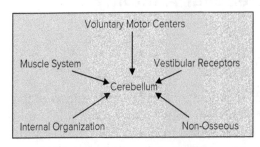

Figure 64: Basic cerebellar afferents

The complex nature of all this input makes the cerebellum responsible for maintaining the synergy of purposeful movement. As a result, it can be referred to as an *"error comparer"* because of its involvement in every aspect of the human neuraxis. It evaluates all incoming signal from muscle and other signals from other areas of the neuraxis, and influences both the conscious and unconscious response to them all. That is a tall order for such a relatively and anatomically small part of the brain, but the cerebellum is uniquely designed to accomplish all these tasks with ease.

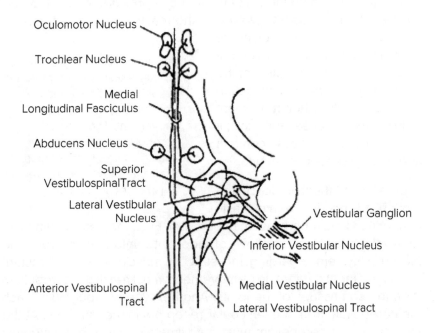

Figure 65: Vestibular afferent and efferent fibers

Anatomical Regions

The cerebellum is phylogenetically divided into three major subdivisions: Archicerebellum, Paleocerebellum and Neocerebellum (Table 18).

1. *Archicerebellum:* ("Archi-" older) The archicerebellum is closely related to the vestibular system. It consists of the uvula, nodulus and flocculus (the joining of the nodulus and flocculus together make up the flocculonodulus). As a result of its early phylogenetic appearance, the archicerebellum is also known as the vestibulocerebellum.

The key words for the archicerebellum are "posture and balance" through the axial skeleton providing for tonus of the extremities. It is the center-most structural support for postural background affording axial stability for shunt stabilization of spurt movement.

Table 18: CEREBELLAR DIVISIONS		
Section	*System*	*Function*
Archicerebellum	Vestibulocerebellum	"Balance" through the axial skeleton providing tonus of the extremities
Paleocerebellum	Spinocerebellum	Controls the "posture and gait" of the more peripheral trunk and girdle muscles
Neocerebellum	Cerebrocerebellum	"Axial control" and "coordination" of skilled learned activity

The vestibulocerebellum has two-way connections (from the medial longitudinal fasciculus of the cervical cord to the vestibular nucleus and from the vestibular nucleus to the vestibulospinal output) with the vestibular nuclei through the medulla (Figure 65). It influences the responses of these nuclei to signals from the vestibular labyrinth. The fastigial nucleus also projects to the gaze centers (eye control through the medial longitudinal fasciculus) of the brain stem in order to coordinate the axial response to visual and auditory input.

Surround Inhibition

If it weren't for the arrangement of the parallel fibers, the Purkinje cells would constantly be stimulated by mossy input, and the paraspinal muscles would be "on" all the time.

* Purkinje cells are the final station for information processing at the level of the cerebellar cortex.

* The principle efferent system of the cerebellum resides in the 4 pairs of cerebellar nuclei.

KEY:

1 = Purkinje cells are the only cerebellar efferents.

2 = Each to a single Purkinje cell.

3 = Intense online activity can be stimulated by inhibition of the Golgi cells.

4 = A glomerulus; each mossy fiber synapses with 500-600 granule cells.

5 = Those Purkinje cells specifically from the vestibulocerebellum.

6 = Other Purkinje cells.

7 = The stimulation by both the mossy and climbing fibers on the Purkinje cells and cerebellar nuclei is modulated by a network of inhibitory cortical interneurons.

MLF = Medial Longitudinal Fasciculus
LVSp = Lateral Vestibulospinal tract
MVSp = Medial Vestibulospinal tract

JMR = Joint Mechanoreceptor input

F = Fastigial nucleus
G = Globose nucleus
E = Emboliform nucleus
D = Dentate nucleus

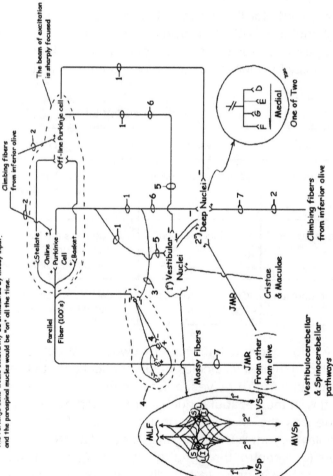

Figure 66: A schematic of the pathways of surround inhibition

The key words for the archicerebellum are "posture and balance" through the axial skeleton providing for tonus of the extremities.

The two-way communication between the vestibular nuclei and the cerebellum are of the most ancient type, with similarities that reach back to the earliest vertebrate nervous systems. It is intricately involved with the function of the cerebellum in general. The vestibulocerebellar and fastigiovestibular pathways play an essential role in the control of limb movements, and vice versa.

2. *Paleocerebellum*: ("Paleo-" long ago; primitive) The paleocerebellum arises as a result of the lateral expansion of the flocculonodulus and consists mostly of the vermis and uvula, and pyramids. It receives sensory input from the periphery and has an output to the spinal cord through descending motor tracts. The paleocerebellum primarily controls movement of the more peripheral trunk and girdle muscles through the reticulospinal tract from the

The key paleocerebellar words involve control of "posture and gait" through the function of the trunk and girdles.

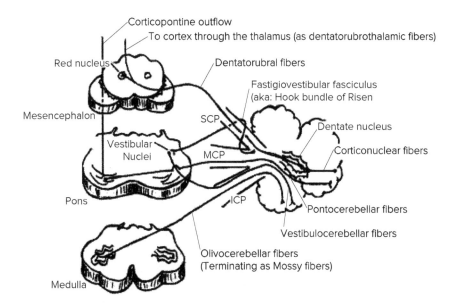

Figure 67: Fiber connections of the cerebellum

contralateral side. Because of its close relationship to the spinal cord, these regions together with the adjacent gracile lobules and intermediate regions of the cerebellar hemispheres are functionally classified as the spinocerebellum.

The spinocerebellum receives direct stimulation from the spine via the spinocerebellar tracts (Figure 71). The key words here are mainly involved with the control of "posture and gait" through the function of the trunk and girdles. It utilizes the globose and emboliform nuclei (the nucleus interpositus) to compare intended and actual movement and correct for the differences.

The vestibular system is also related to the paleocerebellum through the most medial deep cerebellar nuclei—the fastigial nucleus—and sends extensive projections to the vestibular nuclei.

The fastigial nucleus sends excitatory signals to all four vestibular nuclei. The rostral fastigial nucleus fibers project ipsilaterally, while the caudal fastigial nucleus fibers project contralaterally through the uncinate fasciculus or fastigiovestibular fasciculus (aka: Hook Bundle of Risen Russell) to excite the vestibular nucleus (Figure 67).

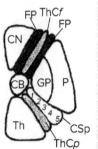

ThCf:	Thalamocortical fibers (to frontal lobe)
FP:	Frontopontine fibers
CN:	Caudate Nucleus
CB:	Corticobulbar fibers
GP:	Globus Pallidus
P:	Putamen
CSp:	Corticospinal fibers [1:Corticonuclear fibers (to head and neck); 2: Corticospinal fibers (to upper limb); 3: Corticospinal fibers (trunk) and Corticorubral fibers; 4: Corticospinal fibers (lower limb); 5: Corticopontine fibers]
Th:	Thalamus
ThCp:	Thalamocortical fibers(to parietal lobe)

Figure 68: Schematic of the fibers that traverse the internal capsule

3. *Neocerebellum:* ("Neo-" newer; recent) Proportional in size to the voluntary motor centers of the cerebrum and like the cerebrum, which overshadows these older portions below it, the neocerebellum, overshadows other aspects of the cerebellum. It is the largest and phylogenetically youngest portion of the cerebellum and consists of the middle vermis and cerebellar

The development of the neocerebellum is closely related to that of the cerebral cortex and to the erect posture of the primates and their ability to resist gravity.

hemispheres. The development of the neocerebellum is closely related to that of the cerebral cortex and to the erect posture of the primates and their ability to resist gravity. The neocerebellum receives extensive spinal input and is functionally classified as part of the spinocerebellum. That part of the neocerebellum that has a very close relationship to the pontine nuclei—the pontocerebellum—receives input from the cerebral cortex and relays modified input back to the cortex via the thalamus through the internal capsule ("ThCf" and "ThCp" in Figure 68), which is very important for connecting cerebral cortex, vital centers and cerebellum. Hence, another name for this division is the "cerebrocerebellum."

The neocerebellum's key words are "axial control" and "coordination" of skilled learned activity through its involvement in planning and initiation of skilled movement. Those skilled movements, initiated by the cerebral motor cortex, are

The neocerebellum's key words are "axial control" and "coordination" of skilled learned activity through its involvement in planning and initiation of skilled movement.

modified by the neocerebellum. The cerebrocerebellum receives a massive feedback input from the contralateral nuclei pontis, via the pontocerebellar fibers (Figure 67) (Table 19).

The archi-, paleo- and neocerebellar designations are overall responsible for the ability to resist gravity and achieve the axial control necessary for upright posture, bipedal balance and gait through trunk and girdle muscles. Without them, the human race would be condemned to constantly hug the ground.

As we shall soon see, the cerebellum does exert control over activities initiated by the stimulation of vestibular receptors (Figure 69).

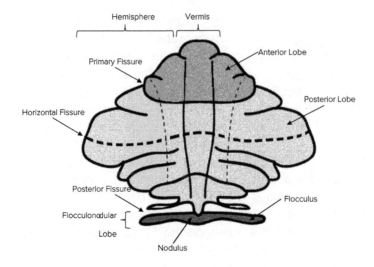

Figure 69:Cerebellar zones, afferents and efferents

		Afferents	Efferents
	Medial	Dorsal spinocerebellar (DSCT) tract	Fastigial nucleus
		Cuneocerebellar (CCT) tract	Reticular formation
		Occipitopontocerebellar (OCT) tract	Vestibular nucleus
ZONE	Intermediate	Dorsal spinocerebellar tract	PCT (from Primary Motor Cortex)
		Cuneocerebellar tract	Interpositus nucleus
		Occipitopontocerebellar tract	Contralateralrubrospinal tract
	Lateral	Occipitopontocerebellar tract	Ipsilateralvestibular nucleus
		Vestibulocerebellar (VCT)tract	Medial and lateral vestibulospinal tracts (MVST&LVST)

Table 19: CEREBELLAR AFFERENTS		
ZONE	INPUT	
	Afferents	Efferents
Medial	DSCT	Fastigial nucleus
	CCT	Reticular formation
	OCT	Vestibular nucleus
Intermediate	DSCT	PCT (from Primary Motor Cortex
	CCT	Interpositus nucleus
	OCT	Contralateral rubrospinal, VA (ventral anterior) / VL (ventral lateral) (both motor related thalamic nuclei), and MI (execution of movement)
Lateral	OCT	Ipsilateral vestibular nucleus
	VCT	MVST & LVST
Refer to Figure 69 for abbreviations.		

Part 2:
Cerebellar Afferents

There are approximately three times as many afferent fibers as efferent fibers emerging from the cerebellum (Figure 70), giving it primary importance as a somatic afferent organ. By far, the largest numbers of projections to the cerebellum are from the cerebral cortex, via the corticopontocerebellar (Figure 68) system through the internal capsule. It provides input to the vital centers of the pons and feedback to the cerebellum. The greatest cerebral representations are from the primary and secondary motor areas and the primary somatosensory areas of the cortex (areas 3, 1, 2, 5 and 7, and the parietal lobe, Broadman's areas 4 and 6, and the frontal lobe).

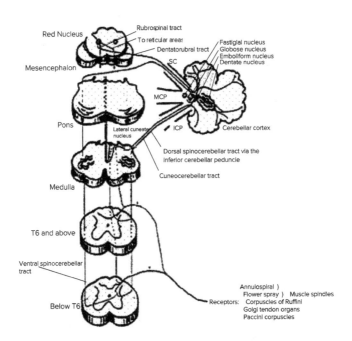

Figure 70: Schematic of cerebellar pathways

These pathways function as relays by which the cerebral cortex acts upon the cerebellar cortex, and vice versa, with completion of the loop via the "ThC*f*" and "ThC*p*" pathways (Figure 68). Arising from a number of discrete neuronal groups in the pons, each of them receives input from a restricted region of the cerebral cortex and projects via the middle cerebellar peduncle to specific areas of the contralateral cerebellar cortex (Figure 67). Their organization, therefore, consists of a point-to-point projection similar to that of the DSCT or CCT (to be discussed ahead). Their precise functional role is unknown, but they may be involved in relaying information regarding cortical motor commands to both the pontine vital centers and the cerebellum.The signals that come to the cerebellum are of two types: mossy fibers (Figure 76) and climbing fibers (Figure 78). The differences between the two are fundamental to understanding their effects on the events of surround inhibition.

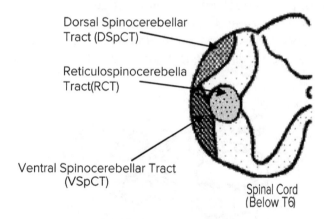

Dorsal Spinocerebellar
Tract (DSpCT)

Reticulospinocerebella
Tract(RCT)

Ventral Spinocerebellar Tract
(VSpCT)

Spinal Cord
(Below T6)

*Figure 71: Dorsal and ventral spinocerebellar
and reticulospinocerebellar tracts*

Mossy Fiber Pathways

Mossy fiber pathways are a well-organized pattern of projections that are found in all parts of the cerebellum. They course upward via the vestibulocerebellar, reticulocerebellar, pontocerebellar, dorsal spinocerebellar, and cuneocerebellar pathways, and give rise to many branches within the granular layer. It is believed that mossy fibers represent the terminations of all fibers that enter the cerebellum from portions of the CNS other than the inferior olivary nucleus, and project to specific regions of the cerebellum:

- Vestibular afferents go to the vestibulocerebellum and fastigial nucleus;

- Spinal afferents go to the spinocerebellum, and globose and emboliform nuclei (as well as the fastigial nucleus);

- Globose, Emboliform and pontocerebellar fibers (from higher centers) go to the cerebrocerebellum with sparse projections to the dentate nucleus.

> Probably the most important aspect of the mossy fiber input to the cerebellum is from the spinocerebellar afferentation.

In other words, nearly all mossy fibers send collaterals to the vestibulocerebellar and spinocerebellar centers, and only a small number of those synapsing with granule cells project to the cerebrocerebellum and send branches to the dentate nucleus via corticonuclear pathways (Figure 67).

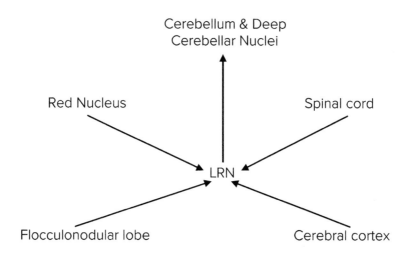

Figure 72: Schematic of pontocerebellar pathways

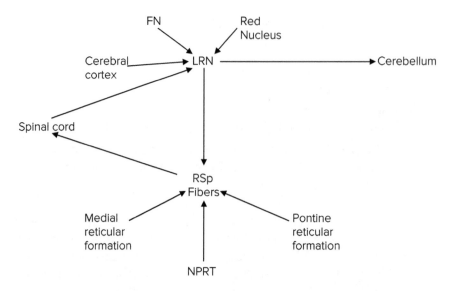

Figure 73: Overview of cerebellar input

Unlike the climbing fibers, mossy fibers do not go directly to the Purkinje cells. Instead, they branch profusely in the white matter (Figure 76), each having multiple (up to 50) swellings that contain round vesicles and synaptic thickenings. These swellings represent moss to the old time neuroanatomists, which is where they got their name. Each swelling, called a "rosette" or "glomerulus", is a synapse of the mossy fiber into the dendrite of a granule cell. Each mossy fiber can have up to 50 of these swellings giving it considerable divergence of its signal.

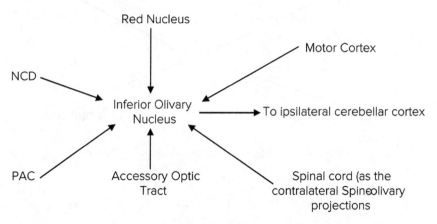

Figure 74: Excitatory input to the inferior olivary nucleus

There are four mossy fiber pathways. They are:

1. Vestibulocerebellar pathways
2. Reticulocerebellar pathways
3. Pontocerebellar pathways
4. Spinocerebellar pathways

> It is very important to recognize that the DSCT generally represents the hind limb while the CCT generally represents the fore limb.

Vestibulocerebellar Pathways

These pathways allow avenues for communication between the various vestibular nuclei (the superior or nucleus of Bechterew, which gives rise to vestibulocerebellar fibers and receives fibers from the cerebellum; the medial, dorsal or the principal nucleus called Schwalbe's Nucleus, which coordinates reflexes of equilibrium and postural gravity; the lateral or nucleus of Deiter, which gives rise to the lateral vestibulospinal tract; and the inferior nucleus, which spawns the anterior vestibulospinal tract) and the deep cerebellar nuclei (Figure 65).

The vestibulocerebellum (Figure 82) receives afferents from the fibers of the cristae as well as those from the maculae. Both give orientation of head motion in space in response to (visual and) auditory stimuli (Figure 66: *A Schematic of the Pathways of Surround Inhibition*).

Some vestibular projections rise through the internal capsule and terminate in the thalamocortical projections of the frontal lobe. Completing the reflex, fibers pass from the frontal and occipital lobes, back through the internal capsule via several descending pathways (Figure 68) to terminate in several areas, one of which is the vestibulocerebellum.

Reticulocerebellar Pathways

Reticulospinal fibers act over wide areas of the cerebellum and deep cerebellar nuclei (Figure 71). They originate from the lateral reticular nucleus (LRN), paramedian reticular nucleus (PRN) in the medulla, and the nucleus reticularis tegmenti

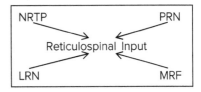

Figure 75: Schematic of reticulocerebellar input

pontis (NRTP) in the pons (Figure 75), and to a lesser degree from the median (magnocellular) reticular formation (MRF). They pass through the inferior cerebellar peduncle to mainly stimulate the vermis of the anterior lobe and perhaps to the flocculonodular lobe of the cerebellum. Some of these fibers may contribute to ventral external arcuate fibers and eventually join the dorsal spinocerebellar tract in the inferior cerebellar peduncle. It may also receive several different types of input, especially from the sensory systems of the spinal cord that pass through the lateral funiculus. The reticulocerebellar pathway is also interconnected with fibers descending from higher motor centers of the extrapyramidal system (Figure 73).

The lateral reticular nucleus (LRN) receives input from the spinal cord (SpC), cerebral cortex (motor areas mostly) (CC), red nucleus (RN), and fastigial nucleus (FN) (Figure 72). These pathways have properties similar to those of the VSCT and RSCT neurons, except that they lack Group I muscle input, are excited by descending vestibulospinal fibers, and typically respond to stimulation of larger areas of body surface.

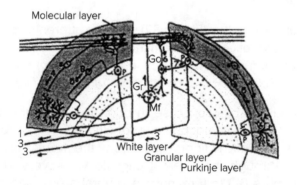

Figure 76: Schematic of Surround Inhibition

1. Mossy fibers stimulate a granule cell (Gr)
2. Beam of parallel activity follows activation of granule cells
3. Activation of on-beam Purkinje cells (P); ("microzone")
4. & 5. Activation of Stellate (S) and Basket cells (B) inhibit off-line Purkinje cells (P)
6. Golgi cells (Go) terminate granule cell activity
7. Intense on-line activity can be sustained by inhibition of Golgi cells

Pontocerebellar Pathways

Most of the pontocerebellar fibers are concerned with the coordination of movements initiated in the motor cortex of the cerebrum. These fibers arise in the frontal, parietal, temporooccipital, and the temporal association areas as well as collaterals of the pyramidal fibers arising in the precentral gyrus, descend through the internal capsule and terminate among the pontine nuclei. These fibers mostly cross to ascend into the cerebellum via the middle cerebellar peduncle. The vast majority of these fibers terminate in the neocerebellar cortex, both of the hemispheres and the vermis. This includes most of the posterior lobe. There is also an overlap with the paleocerebellum of the anterior lobe.

Spinocerebellar Pathways

Probably the most important aspect of the mossy fiber input to the cerebellum, as far as our discussion is concerned, is from the spinocerebellar afferentation (Figure 71). There are two direct pathways from the spinal cord to the cerebellar cortex (Table 20), and each is divided into two sets. They are the:

1. Dorsal spinocerebellar tract (DSCT) and the Cuneocerebellar tract (CCT). Both have forelimb and hind limb components (Table 21), and each subdivides into two functional units.

2. Ventral spinocerebellar tract (VSCT) and the Reticulospinocerebellar tract (RSCT). These paired pathways inform the cerebellar cortex regarding activities of interneurons within the spinal motor centers controlling the hind limbs and forelimbs (Figure 79).

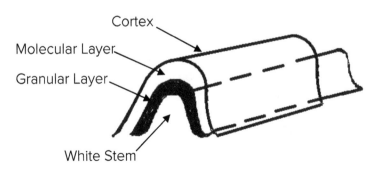

Figure 77: Schematic of the layers of the cerebellar cortex

The DSCT and CCT

The DSCT and CCT pathways convey unconscious proprioception regarding the ipsilateral side of the body. The mesencephalic nucleus of V (trigeminal) conveys such information from the face, and these trigeminocerebellar axons form only a minuscule part of the middle cerebellar peduncle.

Table 20: SPINAL MOTOR AND CEREBELLAR RELATIONSHIPS	
Tract	*From/To*
VSCT	Vestibular nucleus/Cerebellum
RSCT	Reticular system/Cerebellum
Both inform the cerebellar cortex about activities of the interneurons within the spinal motor centers that influence the fore and hind limbs.	

Table 21: FORELIMB AND HIND LIMB PROJECTIONS	
Tract	*From/To*
DSCT	Spinal cord/Cerebellum
CCT	Cuneate nucleus/Cerebellum
Both the DSCT and CCT have fore and hind limb projections.	

The most important point here is that the DSCT and CCT project to the medial and intermediate cerebellar zones (Figure 69). The projections are topographically organized. For instance, there is a representation of the ipsilateral side of the body and head in the anterior lobe. This area, together with the trunk and neck areas are represented in the medial zone. All of this input would be conveyed by both DSCT and CCT fibers. The arm and leg projections are represented in the intermediate zone also, via projections from both

DSCT and CCT fibers. There is a second, larger representation of the ipsilateral side of the body and head in the posterior lobe, and the topographic organization of DSCT and CCT inputs are similar to the anterior lobe. There is a mirror image representation of the body map in the anterior and posterior lobes, such that the head representations lie next to each other.

It is very important to recognize that the DSCT generally represents the hind limb while the CCT generally represents the forelimb. Also, the ipsilateral representation is greater than the contralateral. This will be more clearly important in understanding the effects of each on the more rostral centers they innervate.

Both the DSCT and the CCT convey detailed information from proprioceptors of muscle and exteroceptors responsible for touch and pressure to specific regions of the cerebellar cortex.

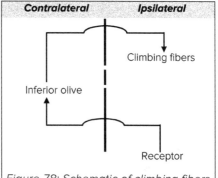

Figure 78: Schematic of climbing fibers as they ascent to the cerebellum

DSCT: The exteroceptive division of the DSCT arises in Clarke's column in the mid-thoracic and upper lumbar spinal cord regions, below the level of T6. These fibers receive input from cutaneous afferent fibers and ascend via the ipsilateral posterolateral funiculus, travel through the inferior cerebellar peduncle to the ipsilaterally located hind limb projection areas in the intermedial part of the anterior lobe and to the gracile lobule.

CCT: The fibers of the CCT originate from the neurons in the lateral cuneate nucleus (Figure 70) and ascend via the inferior cerebellar peduncle to the ipsilaterally located forelimb projection areas adjacent to the dorsal spinocerebellar termination areas.

A majority of the proprioceptive neurons come from the muscle spindle afferents (Group Ia and to a lesser degree Group II) and from Golgi tendon organ afferents (Group Ib), which signal muscle length and tension, respectively.

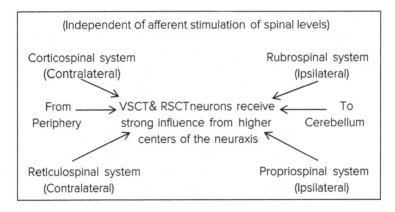

Figure 79: The descending pathways that influence the ventral spinocerebellar (VSCT) &reticulospinocerebellar (RSCT) tracts

Each individual DSCT and CCT neuron receives input from only a few closely related muscles (organized via homologous columns) and provides detailed information regarding muscle activity to the cerebellum. A small group of DSCT and CCT neurons relay information from joint mechanoreceptors for more organized muscle function. Also, many proprioceptive DSCT and CCT neurons receive weak background excitation from high threshold muscle afferents.

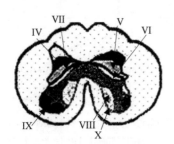

Figure 80: Laminar distribution according to Rexed

The exteroceptive DSCT and CCT fibers follow a similar course and terminate in the same region as the proprioceptive DSCT and CCT axons. The signals carried by exteroceptive DSCT and CCT neurons originate primarily from touch and hair receptors in the skin. An individual DSCT and CCT neuron receives input from a small area of skin, which means that these neurons can provide detailed information regarding touch probably for learned defensive response.

VSCT and RSCT

The VSCT takes its origin from the bordered cells of Rexed V, VI, and VII (Figure 80). They decussate and ascend in the anterolateral funiculus and enter the cerebellum through the contralateral superior cerebellar peduncle. They terminate bilaterally in the spinocerebellum, most densely on the ipsilateral hind limb region with fibers from the DSCT termination.

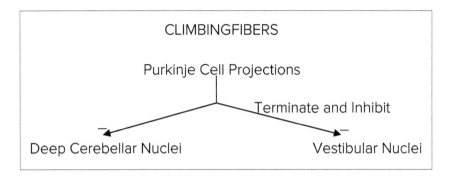

Figure 81: Schematic of cerebellar fibers descending to two of the major centers for surround inhibition

The RSCT originate from the neurons at the base of the posterior spinal horn. The nerves ascend ipsilaterally in the posterior funiculus and enter the cerebellum via both the inferior and superior cerebellar peduncles. Once in the cerebellum, the RSCT axons terminate widely throughout the fore limb and hind limb portions of the spinocerebellum on both sides.

All the afferent systems that provide mossy fiber projections to the cerebellum also send afferents to the entire contralateral cerebellum by way of the inferior olivary nucleus, which gives rise to the climbing fiber system.

The nerves of the VSCT and RSCT receive complex patterns of peripheral input that seem related to the signals received by interneurons of the spinal motor pathways. Many VSCT and RSCT neurons are directly excited by Group I muscle afferents, predominately those originating from Golgi tendon organs, which carry information regarding muscle tone. An individual neuron typically receives such excitation form a large group of leg muscles involved in a particular pattern of movement. VSCT and RSCT neurons also receive input from multisynaptic spinal pathways that are activated by cutaneous and high threshold muscle afferent fibers.

The Inferior Olivary Nucleus

The inferior olivary nucleus receives excitatory input from the spinal cord (SpC) via several afferent pathways from cutaneous and muscle receptors, motor cortex, red nucleus (RN), nucleus of Cajal and Darkschewitz (NCD), periaqueductal gray (PAG) matter and the accessory optic

> The inferior olive may have to do with the comparison of intended versus ongoing movement.

tract (AOT). The spinal neurons projecting to one inferior olive are located on the side contralateral to the olive, which is ipsilateral to the region of cerebellar cortex to which its climbing fibers project (Figure 74).

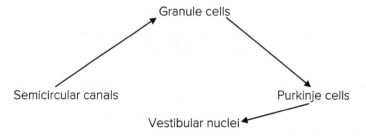

An inhibitory circuit that parallels semicircular canal input to the vestibular nuclei.It modulates the vestibulospinal reflex.

Figure 82: The shortest circuit through the vestibulocerebellum

The inferior olivary nucleus is the sole source of climbing fibers to the cerebellum and is involved in exciting motor coordination. There are two inputs to the inferior olive. The first is an ascending afferent tract from the spinal cord via spino-olivary projections (which carries somatosensory input). The other afferent tract descends via the uncrossed primary motor cortex (MI) through the cortico-olivary tract.

The inferior olive may have to do with the comparison of intended versus ongoing movement. Such correction information is conveyed to the intermediate zone of the cerebellum.

Climbing Fiber Pathways

All the afferent systems that provide mossy fiber projections to the cerebellum (somatosensory, visual, auditory, vestibular, and corticopontocerebellar) also send afferents to the entire contralateral cerebellum by way of the inferior olivary nucleus, which gives rise to the climbing fiber system (Figure 70). These long and slender fibers send collaterals to the contralateral deep cerebellar nuclei via the inferior cerebellar peduncle and then "climb" up and, like ivy, entwining and synapsing all over the dendrites of the Purkinje cell. This is where their name comes from—from their characteristic climb among the dendritic ramifications of Purkinje cells like a vine on a trellis.

Each terminal climbing fiber branch often makes 300 to 500 individual excitatory synapses upon a single Purkinje cell. Each Purkinje cell, however, receives the input from only one climbing fiber axon. Therefore, when the climbing fiber fires, there is massive, synchronous and extremely strong depolarization of the Purkinje cell. In fact, the synaptic connection between the climbing fiber and the Purkinje cell is one of the most powerful in the nervous system.

> All special sensory input arrives in the cerebellum via tectocerebellar fibers.

Climbing fibers are "lazy" (but strong), causing Purkinje stimulation at the rate of about one per second. Nonetheless, stimulation of the climbing fiber significantly alters the responsiveness of the Purkinje cell to subsequent parallel fiber stimulation for periods up to several hours. This stimulation causes a reduction in Purkinje cell sensitivity to parallel fiber stimulation, an effect known as long-term depression (LTD). Because Purkinje cells are inhibitory, the LTD of Purkinje cells disinhibits neurons in the cerebellar nuclei increasing their basal firing rate and rendering them more sensitive to other excitatory signals, i.e., collaterals from mossy fibers and climbing fibers.

> Each of the signals from the Purkinje cells that terminate in the deep cerebellar nuclei is inhibitory.

Special Sense Afferents

All special sensory input arrives in the cerebellum via tectocerebellar fibers. The tectum of the mesencephalon has been shown to be the center for visual and auditory

> In general, the Purkinje cells modulate (inhibit) excitatory relay neurons that project to other parts of the CNS involved in motor and autonomic control.

reflexes, thus this pathway has to do with the coordination of the motor portion of these reflexes. It has been suggested that the tectocerebellar route is the most important pathway linking auditory impulses to the cerebellum. Visual impulses may have other routes such as the tectopontocerebellar or occipitopontocerebellar pathways.

Zones of the Cerebellum and Distribution of Fibers

The various cerebellar afferents distribute to four different zones of the cerebellum. These are the 1) medial zone, 2) intermediate zone, 3) lateral zone, and 4) flocculonodular zone (or lobe). (Figure 37)

1. Olivocerebellar fibers—distribute to the entire cerebellum

2. Cuneocerebellar (CCT) fibers—distribute to the medial and intermediate zones

3. Dorsal spinocerebellar (DSCT) fibers—distribute to the medial and intermediate zones

4. Pontocerebellar fibers—distribute to the intermediate and lateral zones

   a. Those pontine gray neurons that project to the intermediate zone of the cerebellum receive their corticopontine input from the primary motor cortex (area 4)

   b. Those pontine grey neurons that project to the lateral zone of the cerebellum receive their corticopontine input from posterior parietal cortex and are more involved in planning the motor act than in execution of the program.

5. Vestibulocerebellar fibers—(arise from the vestibular ganglion and nuclei) distribute primarily to the flocculonodular lobe

Deep Cerebellar Nuclei

Each of the four different cerebellar zones—the medial, lateral, intermediate and flocculonodular zones—contains Purkinje cells which project their axons to different deep cerebellar nuclei (Table 22).

Table 22: DEEP CEREBELLAR AFFERENTS/EFFERENTS		
Nuclei	*Input/ From*	*Function*
Dentate	Lateral Zone/ Olivo- & Ponto- Cerebellar Tracts	Planning info
Interpositus	Intermediate Zone/Olivo- & Ponto- Cerebellar Tracts & CCT	Primary motor cortex, DSCT
Fastigial	Medial Zone/DSCT, CCT & Olive	
Vestibular	Flocculonodular Zone	Balance

The most lateral deep cerebellar nucleus, the dentate, receives its Purkinje cell input from the lateral zone of the cerebellum. This lateral zone of the cerebellum receives its input from olivocerebellar and pontocerebellar fibers carrying planning information from the posterior parietal area. The interpositus nucleus (globose and emboliform) receives its Purkinje cell input from the intermediate zone of the cerebellum, which receives its input from olivocerebellar and pontocerebellar fibers carrying information from primary motor cortex (area 4) and from the DSCT and CCT. The Purkinje cells that innervate the medially located fastigial nucleus lie in the medial zone of the cerebellum and receive input from the DSCT, CCT and the olive.

Purkinje cells in the flocculonodular zone (or lobe) also need a deep nucleus. They terminate in the

- Cerebellar lesions result in ipsilateral motor incoordination.
- Lesions of inferior cerebellar peduncle are ipsilateral problems.
- The inferior olive projects to the contralateral cerebellum, therefore lesions of the inferior olive are seen as contralateral motor incoordination.

209

vestibular nuclei, which we can consider to be a "surrogate" deep cerebellar nucleus. These Purkinje cells that are destined for the vestibular nuclei travel in the inferior cerebellar peduncle (along with the fibers from the vestibular nerve and nuclei that are entering the cerebellum).

Each of the signals from the Purkinje cells that terminate in the deep cerebellar nuclei is inhibitory. The deep cerebellar nuclei also receive excitatory inputs from the collaterals of both mossy and climbing fibers as they pass through the deep white matter on their way to the overlying cerebellar cortex. The summation of the inhibitory (Purkinje cell) and excitatory (mossy and climbing fiber) inputs to the deep cerebellar and vestibular nuclei (Figure 81) determines their CIS, or the quality of excitatory or inhibitory output signal to the other parts of the brain.

Part 3:
Cerebellar Efferents

To enhance functional display, cerebellar organization is primarily important. Its cortex is specifically arranged to adapt to its unique functional requirements. First, the cerebellum must be able to exert its modulatory influence over the musculature of the entire body. This requires a single impulse to spread over, and activate large areas of cortex. Second, the influence of the cerebellum must be able to influence, enhance and perpetuate action potentials. Therefore, the action potentials must be able to reactivate the same areas in the cortex from which they originally arose. This is what it means to be homologously-related.

> There are enough parallel fibers in the adult cerebellum to encircle the earth almost two and a half times.

The cerebellar cortex is arranged into three layers: outer or molecular layer, the middle or Purkinje cell layer, and the inner or granular layer (Figures 76 & 77).

Molecular Layer

The molecular layer is almost entirely taken up by Purkinje cell dendrites, parallel fibers, supporting neuroglial cells and blood vessels. In the adult, the cerebellum contains more than 100,000 kilometers of parallel fibers—enough to encircle the earth nearly two and one half times. Further, the molecular layer is the home of the stellate and basket cells (Table 23). They are the only interneurons in the molecular layer, and both of them are inhibitory. Both make contact with parallel fibers (the only excitatory input to both the stellate and basket cells) and both synapse on the most adjacent five to eight

> The cerebellar tissues must be oxygenated at all times in order for the most oxygen sensitive tissues—the Purkinje cells—to survive.

Purkinje cells. However, a single basket cell can synapse with some 250 Purkinje cells.

Table 23: CEREBELLAR SPECIALTY CELLS	
Layer	Contents
Molecular	Stellate and Basket cells
Purkinje	Purkinje cell bodies
Granular	Granular and Golgi cell bodies

Purkinje layer

The Purkinje layer is also known as the "piriform" layer. It contains the largest and most oxygen sensitive tissues in the entire neuraxis— the Purkinje cells. They also compose the largest dendritic trees in the neuraxis, which are oriented at right angles to the parallel fibers. Each Purkinje cell is penetrated by and receives synaptic contact from about 200,000 parallel fibers, each one making up successive, single synapses upon the dendritic spines of about 400 Purkinje cells. The display of this massive input will be discussed in a moment.

Granular layer

The granular layer contains around 10 billion (1×10^{11}) granule cells. That is more neurons than in both cerebral hemispheres combined. Each of the granule cells has a body the size of a red blood cell. Axons of granule cells penetrate to the molecular layer where they divide into "T" shaped parallel fibers. They make excitatory synapses with Purkinje cells.

The granule cells receive mossy fiber input from all sources except the inferior olivary nucleus; those go elsewhere. Before reaching the cerebellar cortex, the mossy fibers, which are excitatory in nature, give off collateral branches to the deep cerebellar nuclei (Figure 66: *A Schematic of the Pathways of Surround Inhibition*).

Granular cells have long axons that pass dorsally through the granular and Purkinje cell layers to reach the molecular layer of the cerebellar cortex, where they bifurcate and run parallel to the long axis of the folium (Figure 76). They travel at right angles to the dendrites of the Purkinje cells. Each of these parallel fibers synapses upon and excites the dendritic spines of numerous Purkinje cells, but the synaptic effect of a single parallel fiber upon a Purkinje cell is extremely weak. However, many mossy fiber-granule cell connections stimulate lots of parallel fibers to fire rapidly and together at about one cycle per second. In contrast to those lazy climbing fibers that fire about one time per second, mossy fibers have a profound simultaneous and rapid display of about 50-100 times per second with the Purkinje cells firing at about the same frequency.

Cerebellar cortical projections to the lateral vestibular nucleus serve to regulate the activation of the descending spinal motor apparatus.

In addition to the climbing fiber and mossy fiber-granule cell-parallel fiber input to the Purkinje cells, which are excitatory, there are other inputs to the Purkinje cell that are inhibitory. The first of these cells is the granule cell layer and is called a Golgi cell. Compared to the many millions of small granule cells, there are relatively few Golgi cells and they are much larger than granule cells. The dendrites of the Golgi cells lie in the molecular layer and are excited by the parallel fibers of granule cells. The axon of the Golgi cell enters into a complex arrangement with the mossy fiber terminal-granule cell dendrite (the glomerulus) such that the Golgi cell axon inhibits the mossy fiber-granule cell relay. This is called feedback inhibition, because the Golgi cell inhibits information that is coming into the cerebellar circuitry. Because of the wide spread of Golgi cell dendrites and axons within the cerebellar cortex, their actions further restrict the focus of excitation produced by mossy fiber action and reinforces the surrounding zone of inhibition.

The parallel fibers of granule cells (which travel in the molecular layer) also excite the dendrites of basket cells. Both the dendrites and somas of the basket cells lie in the molecular layer. These dendrites, like those of Purkinje cells, lie in a plane that is transverse to the long axes of the folia. The axons of basket cells also run in this plane (transverse to the long axis of the folia) and terminate on the somas of the Purkinje cells. The inhibition of Purkinje cells by the basket cell axons is called feed-forward inhibition. Another way to look at these types of inhibition is whether the inhibiting cell is acting on an "earlier" or "later" cell in the cerebellar circuitry.

Cerebellar Output

There is only one set of fibers leaving the cerebellar cortex. These are all the axons of Purkinje cells that pass through the molecular layer of the cerebellar cortex to reach the white, medullary core of the folium. Continuing in the white substance, most of these axons end in one of the four central nuclei. Few leave the cerebellum directly. In general, the Purkinje cells modulate (inhibit) excitatory relay neurons that project to other parts of the CNS involved in motor and autonomic control.

All cerebellar cortical output is conducted centrally by the Purkinje cell axons. Under normal circumstances, Purkinje cells discharge rhythmically, so that both excitatory and inhibitory modulation of their baseline activity can vary the amount of inhibition produced in their target neurons in the deep cerebellar or vestibular nuclei (Figure 66: *A Schematic of the Pathways of Surround Inhibition*).

Cerebellar cortical projections to the lateral vestibular nucleus serve to regulate the activation of the descending spinal motor apparatus. Too much signal provides for quite severe paraspinal muscle spasm and too little allows for the breakdown of shunt stabilization for spurt activity, leading to production of by-products of tissue destruction, and chemical nociceptive elements causing sensitization, with a compromise of spinal curves as a result of chemically induced nociception, culminating in the expression of a degenerative posture.

Next, we will discuss the vascular system that provides the building blocks that make up the essential components for tissue reparation—oxygen and other nutrients necessary for tissue repair.

Part 4:
Cerebellar Vascularity

There appears to be an obvious link between the head and neck, as part of the nerve supply to the head comes from the neck. The posterior cranial fossa is innervated by the upper cervical nerves and the sympathetic trunk. These nerves enter the posterior cranial fossa via the foramen magnum, hypoglossal canal, and jugular foramen. The

As a result of embryonic differentiation, segmental afferentation is projected to and efferentation is received from those centers of the neuraxis that are homologously related. The result is functional facilitation and functional inhibition when each is physiologically necessary.

nerves to the dura which enter the cranial cavity via the hypoglossal canal and jugular foramen are derived from anterior rami of the first and second cervical nerves and from the superior cervical ganglion. Some of the sensory nerve fibers in the dura mater may influence pain. Another idea is that other sensory nerve fibers in the dura mater may be concerned with pressure regulation and that they constitute the afferent side of a reflex neural pathway that controls blood flow to the capillary beds of the choroid plexus. Due to the close proximity of blood vessels, these nerves may be more closely associated with vascular headache and migraine (Figure 83).

The flow of blood is the lifeline to any tissue. In order for it to be effective, it must be consistent and uninterrupted. Blood carries the essential components for normal tissue respiration. Without an adequate blood supply, some tissues die in a matter of seconds. This is especially true of the cerebellum because of its primary demand for oxygen. The cerebellar tissues must be oxygenated at all times in order for the most oxygen sensitive tissues—the Purkinje cells—to survive. Other tissues may last up to only a few minutes without oxygen before dying.

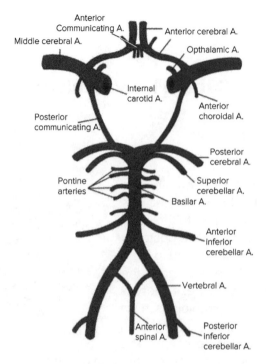

Figure 83: More caudal portion of the Circle of Willis (From Gray's Anatomy)

Arterial Supply

A properly functioning vascular system should function flawlessly to deliver nutrients to the tissues of the body, particularly to those of the cranium. A normal blood flow is unperceivable, but a distention of the vessels sends nociceptive signals to more rostral centers and if they reach the conscious cortex they are recognized as pain and we say "ouch".

The process of keeping pain under control is one of the reasons for this chapter. It is the functional signal of large

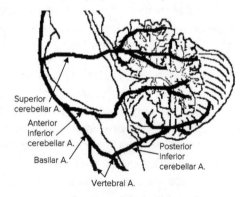

Figure 84: Main cerebellar arteries (From Gray's Anatomy)

diameter axons from joint mechanical receptors that presynaptically inhibits nociceptive inputs in the dorsal horn of the cord that keep pain from being perceived. Modulation is the key to a normal and healthy nervous system.

The cerebellum gets its oxygenated blood from the anastomosis of the two vertebral arteries inside the foramen magnum, which form the basilar artery (Figures 83 and 84). Prior to the anastomosis and along their intracranial course, the vertebral arteries give off several branches: 1) the anterior and posterior spinal arteries, which go along the ventral side of the medulla and spinal cord, and to the spinal cord along its dorsal roots, and 2) the posterior inferior cerebellar artery which usually begins just below the union where the two vertebral arteries form the basilar artery. The posterior inferior cerebellar artery (PICA) nourishes the lateral medulla, most of the inferior half of the cerebellum and the inferior vermis (Figure 83).

Interestingly, the brain itself is insensitive to pain.

The word "learning" as used here, refers to the ability to modify motor responses or sequences in order to adapt the responses to a new situation or changes in surrounding conditions.

The basilar artery ascends along the pons and terminates by dividing into the posterior cerebral arteries. Along its course, the basilar artery gives rise—among other arteries—to the anterior inferior cerebellar artery (AICA), which supplies the inferior lateral pons, the middle cerebellar peduncle and a strip of the cerebellum between the territories of the PICA and the SCA, including the flocculus.

Just prior to its termination into the posterior cerebral artery, the basilar artery also gives rise to the superior cerebellar artery (SCA) that supplies the upper lateral pons and the superior cerebellar

The cerebellum is intimately connected to the vital centers of the pons through the homologous pathways.

peduncle along with most of the superior half of the cerebellar hemisphere, as well as the corpora quadrigemini, pineal body and the choroid plexus of the third ventricle, and the deep cerebellar nuclei and the superior vermis (Figure 84).

Venous Network

Generally speaking, the veins that drain all the brain areas terminate in the dural sinuses. They are classified as internal and external cerebral and cerebellar veins. Since the latter are of our particular interest, it is essential that we understand the avenues of venous drainage of the cerebellum.

Simply, there are two cerebellar veins, one the superior and the other the inferior. The former allows the passage of venous blood into the straight sinus, internal cerebral veins, transverse sinus and superior petrosal sinus. The latter directs its drainage into the transverse, superior petrosal and occipital sinuses.

> Functionally, the vital centers influence such things as the flow of saliva as a result of certain smells or tastes, or the cessation of saliva or dryness as a result of emotions.

There are other lesser caliber veins—the emissary veins and diploic veins—to equalize pressure inside the cranium. The emissary veins connect the intra- and extracranial veins while the diploic veins form venous plexuses between the inner and outer tables of the skull. They both finally drain into the sinuses of the cranium.

Cerebellar Vascular Modulation

The dura of the posterior cranial fossa is supplied by the vagus nerve (X) and the upper cervical nerves. There are also interconnecting fibers between the upper cervical nerves and the hypoglossal nerve forming the ansa cervicales which

> Of all the fibers that exit the cerebrum through the internal capsule, about 10 percent go the muscles while the other 90 percent go to autonomic centers.

also supply this territory. The ascending branches of the meningeal rami (otherwise known as the sinuvertebral nerve) of the 2nd and 3rd cervical levels extend through the foramen magnum to supply the dura mater of the posterior cranial fossa.

There are descriptions of the lower cranial nerves supplying the posterior cranial fossa. All the bulbar nerves are very closely connected to each other, and all have links with the trigeminal nucleus. The vagus nerve has its superior ganglion sitting in the jugular foramen. It communicates with the nearby sympathetic trunk and with the facial (VII), glossopharyngeal (IX), and accessory (XI) nerves. The central processes of the superior vagal ganglion cells probably end in the spinal nuclei of the trigeminal (V) nerve. The IX is very closely related anatomically to the vagus (X) nerve. There are a few general somatic afferent impulses from the meninges of the posterior cranial fossa that end in the spinal tract and nucleus of the trigeminal (V) nerve. The hypoglossal (XII) nucleus is also interconnected to the vagal (X), glossopharyngeal (IX) and trigeminal (V) sensory nuclei, probably through the reticular formation.

Pain inside the cranium—also known as a headache—actually comes from post-stenotic vascular dilation.

Through the pathways described in parts two and three, we can see that the fibers of cerebellar input and output are designed to provide for optimal function and maintain optimal response to the periphery. If that climate gets disturbed or the capacity for response is exceeded for various reasons, the neuraxis compromises leading to structural and functional problems discussed next.

Aside from the concept of homologous columns, the cortex is unable to distinguish the precise area from which a nociceptive impulse arises.

Interestingly, the brain itself is insensitive to pain. The only structures of the cranium able to sense pain are the scalp and its blood vessels, head and neck muscles, great venous sinuses, arteries of the meninges, larger cerebral arteries, pain-sensitive fibers of cranial nerves V, IX, and X, and parts of the dura mater at the base of the brain. Irritation of these structures can cause headache.

Pain inside the cranium—also known as a headache—actually comes from post-stenotic vascular dilation, which causes depolarization of nociceptive receptors in the web-like network of nerves around the blood vessels called the perivascular plexus. The stretch of the blood vessels causes a discharge of the nociceptive receptors and pain can be perceived along the trigeminal and upper cervical pathways.

As a result of embryonic differentiation, segmental afferentation is projected to and efferentation is received from those centers of the neuraxis that are homologously related.

219

Blood vessels are the containers that transport blood and blood substrates. They are made up of smooth muscle fibers with contractile properties. Both the postganglionic and nociceptive fibers are type C. They both have the same diameter and degree of myelination, and therefore the same threshold. Therefore, when one discharges, an adjacent one of similar type also has the potential to discharge as a result of "empathic transmission" or "cross talk."

There is a neurological link between the upper cervical nerves and the sensory fibers of the trigeminal nerve, which receives nociceptive information from the face and other pain sensitive structures in the head. As the upper three cervical nerves enter the dorsal columns, via the dorsal root ganglion, their fibers synapse with the descending fibers of the spinal trigeminal nucleus which descends within the spinal cord caudally to the level of C3 (and some texts say as far as C7).

The signals mingle in the interneuronal synapses of the spinal cord and travel up to the cerebral cortex. Aside from the concept of homologous columns, the cortex is unable to distinguish the precise area from which a nociceptive impulse arises, so information from the cervical spinal nerves is perceived to be indiscernible from trigeminal impulses. This is the idea of referred pain.

Part 5:
Cerebellar Modulation of Vital Centers

Recall that the cerebellum and pons are both derived from the same type of embryonic tissue. That means that whatever happens to one tissue will be felt by every related tissue—another aspect of homologous columns.

The summation of sensory input to more rostral centers is dependent upon the quality and quantity of joint motion perceived by various types of receptors.

Not only are the normal signals from joint mechanical receptors necessary for modulating nociceptive signals, but also for managing the signals that influence the centers for vital functions. Some of the most important signals for this control come from the reticular formation.

The reticular system is responsible for those aspects of neurologic influence that modulate vital functions. It permeates the entire brainstem and fills the spaces between cranial nerve nuclei and olivary bodies and between ascending and descending fiber tracts with groups of neurons and axons.

Statistically, there is more pathological expression resulting from deafferentation than from frank tissue damage.

Many neurons of the reticular formation have autonomic functions. These neurons are scattered throughout the pons and medulla, which explains their close connections with somatic cranial nerve nuclei.

Because of its influence on the spinal reflex arcs, the reticular formation plays a large role in keeping muscle tone adequate for walking, standing, and maintaining equilibrium. It is composed of two general parts.

The ascending reticular system is essentially important in maintaining the state of consciousness, the state of attentive alertness, and the rhythm of wakefulness and sleep.

The descending reticular pathways are said to be influenced by the cerebral cortex, particularly those fibers from the frontal cortex, by the cerebellum, and by the basal ganglia—all part of the corticobulbar fibers of the extrapyramidal system.

The learning of complex motor tasks and sequencing along with motor plasticity are two functions that involve the olivocerebellar climbing fiber system.

The reticular formation receives afferent input from, and sends efferent impulses to the spinal cord, cranial nerve nuclei, cerebellum, and the cerebrum. One group of reticular formation nuclei influences spinal motor action as well as autonomic functions via descending fibers. Another group of reticular formation nuclei, particularly those located in the midbrain, project to more rostrally located centers through the thalamus and subthalamus. These centers also receive input from the spine, nucleus of the solitary tract, vestibular and cochlear nuclei, and optic and olfactory systems. They also give input to widespread areas of the cerebral cortex.

The cerebellum is intimately connected to the vital centers of the pons through their homologous pathways. Specifically, the cerebellopontine signals are received by the pons via the middle cerebellar peduncle while the corticopontine pathways traverse the internal capsule on their way to the pons. Other aspects of this same loop (pontocerebellar and pontothalamic pathways, respectively) originate in the pons and midbrain. The vital centers also receive input from the spinal cord via the contralateral spinothalamic and spinoreticular pathways.

With sufficient spatial and temporal summation, the neurons reach threshold resulting in afferentation of more rostral centers, resulting in a functional display of about 10% of the cerebral outflow; the other 90% goes to autonomic centers.

Functionally, the vital centers influence such things as the flow of saliva as a result of certain smells or tastes, or the cessation of saliva or dryness as a result of emotions. Other of the vital centers control blood pressure, heart and pulse rate, inspiration and expiration, control or coordination of intestinal movement, swallowing, vomiting and retching, and oral movements concerned with the uptake or food, such as chewing, licking, and sucking.

Pontocerebellar fibers that convey information from the posterior parietal (higher motor planning) area of the cortex terminate within the lateral zone of the cerebellum. Those that convey information from the primary motor cortex (MI, or area 4) terminate within the intermediate zone. They are topographically organized and overlap with DSCT and CCT fibers.

Of all the fibers that exit the cerebrum through the internal capsule, about 10 percent go the muscles while the other 90 percent go to autonomic centers throughout the brainstem and cerebellum, including the vital centers of the reticular formation in one way or another.

In general, the signals that enter the cerebellum from various sources generally exit through the Purkinje cells to modulate the vestibular nuclei and those centers postsynaptic to the cerebellopontine tracts. These are the centers of vital function that are intimately connected to cerebellar function.

The point is that whatever happens to the cerebellum will have a modulatory effect upon the functions of the vital centers and vice versa, and ultimately both areas have an influence upon the character of autonomic expression.

Part 6:
Cerebellar Lesions

As we have seen from the preceding pages, the cerebellum is quite dependent upon the information it receives in order to modify both muscular and autonomic function. The secret to accurate functional somatic and autonomic display is sufficient quality and quantity of afferent input.

The effects of dysafferentation can be seen during a neurological examination that incorporates functional testing.

The summation of sensory input to more rostral centers is dependent upon the quality and quantity of joint motion perceived by various types of receptors. In order to fully stimulate the more rostral homologue, the more caudal one must be brought to threshold consistent with the physiological movement of the segment. This is what we call functional motion. Only functional expression will cause a physiologic display. Anything other than functional motion should be considered pathological, leading to a dysfunctional display as perceived through neurological testing.

One way to express proper cerebellar activity is to discuss its metabolic parameters. In the last chapter, we said that—since the two areas are homologously related through the metencephalon—the cerebellum has influence over pontine centers for vital controls and pontine function is displayed in the cerebellum. We said that the cerebellum can modify the vital functions depending upon the demands placed upon them by somatic structures requiring a like response in the centers that provide control of the autonomic expression of those segments.

Coupled Motion

As a result of embryonic differentiation, segmental afferentation is projected to and efferentation is projected from those centers of the neuraxis that are homologously related. The result is functional facilitation and functional

Many learned responses are reflexive and many are pre-programmed in areas called central pattern generators (CPGs).

inhibition of the homologously-related muscles when each is required for normal physiological expression.

The most significant afferentation to the CNS is from the joints of the skeleton through joint mechanical receptors. The non-osseous receptors of the more rostral spinal segments hold the highest priority in the entire human nervous system, and the influence decreases as; you go more caudally. However, the spinal segments generally have more influence upon higher parts of the neuraxis than do the more peripheral segments. Further, the upper extremities have a greater influence upon more rostral centers than do the lower extremities. Finally, the more rostral aspects of the upper extremity are more neurologically significant than the more caudal aspects of the same extremity.

When segments move, the receptors that pick up that modality are discharged. With sufficient spatial and temporal summation, the neurons reach threshold and send an afferent

Properly integrated postural mechanisms are the motor expression of appropriately organized and adequately facilitated rostral centers.

signal to more rostral centers resulting in a functional display of about 10% of the cerebral outflow; the other 90% goes to autonomic centers. To say it another way: With few exceptions, 10% of every input received by the CNS—including the receiving, processing and integrating information—ultimately finds expression in contraction of a muscle for either purposeful motion or postural control. The other 90% of cerebral outflow never reaches the muscles, but instead is routed to autonomic centers. That is, both physiological motion and dysfunctional display lead to some kind of expression—both structural and autonomic—with the former being well-expressed and the latter being pathological.

Understanding the normal character of cerebellar display helps realize that which is pathological. This can be done easily with practice and study.

Statistically, there is more pathological expression resulting from deafferentation than from frank tissue damage. Damage to the cerebellum in the form of a pathological lesion or deafferentation produce a variety of motor disturbances. Depending on the location and extent of the insult, the effects occur singly or in combination with other expressions. Most cerebellar disorders lead to the abnormal performance of a motor task rather than to a loss of motor function or a paresis.

Throughout this entire chapter, the main point is that the cerebellum is a grid work of "beams" that respond specifically to certain sequences of events in the input and in turn produce sequences of signals in the output. The essence of the various inputs and outputs must be synchronous relative to all others. Well, if the input barrage from the joint mechanical receptors is dysfunctional or deafferentated for whatever reason, then the resulting autonomic and structural display will be pathological.

...no matter what nerves go where, the effects of dysfunctional joint motion allow the expression of what should otherwise be inhibited.

Here is an example of physiological and pathological cerebellar expression: The Purkinje cells of the cerebellar vermis (paleocerebellum; spinocerebellum)—which is also related to the vestibulocerebellum through the fastigial nucleus—can depress the activity of neurons throughout the vestibular nuclei either by direct inhibition or by inhibiting the discharge of neurons in the fastigial nucleus, thereby decreasing the excitatory activity reaching the vestibular neurons via fastigiovestibular pathways (Figure 66: *A Schematic of the Pathways of Surround Inhibition*)—an example of dysfacilitation or surround inhibition.

Although the paleocerebellum has a widespread action on the vestibular nuclei, it receives only a modest amount of direct vestibular afferent input, plus some vestibular information relayed via indirect pathways. Much more important input arrives in the paleocerebellum via the spinocerebellar tracts. It therefore seems probable that the principle action of the paleocerebellum on the vestibular system is to regulate vestibular activity in response to input of information from the spinal cord. One such action, as mentioned earlier, is the degree of tone in the muscles that support the intrinsic muscles of the spine.

On the other hand, let's say that trauma impacts a spinal segment. Part of the traumatic display is an increase in tone in the intrinsic spinal muscles that limits the segment's full excursion through its physiological range of motion. This leads to inappropriate stimulation of the joint mechanical receptors with a high probability of facilitation of those areas that should be inhibited, and inhibition of those areas that should be facilitated. By definition, these sequencing errors represent problems that alter the normal physiological expression and should always be considered pathological. For the purposes of our discussion, we call these sequencing problems "dysafferentation" or "dyscoupling," i.e., dysfunctional afferent input to more rostral centers.

The effects of dysafferentation can be seen during a neurological examination that incorporates functional testing. Nevertheless, the expression of that dysafferentation leads to an inability to physiologically facilitate the mossy and/or climbing fibers, leading to the inability to adequately stimulate Purkinje function. This leads to the expression of that action the Purkinje cells would have otherwise inhibited. Without properly working control mechanisms in place, the lateral vestibulospinal tract could cause such fierce muscle contraction and resultant extension response so powerful that it could break bone.

> Generally, although a person may have symptoms below the level of T6, the more rostral centers influence what happens in the more caudal centers.

The learning of complex motor tasks and sequencing along with motor plasticity are two functions that involve the olivocerebellar climbing fiber system. The word "learning," as used here, refers to the modification of motor responses or sequences in order to adapt the responses to a new situation or changes in surrounding conditions. This may represent enhanced physiological expression as well as well as it can pathology.

Much of the somatic motor function is semiautomatic. We do not consciously "think" about all the motor movements involved when we reach for an object. For example, we do not "consciously" extend each finger to grasp the object or consciously adjust the tone in postural muscles to maintain balance. Our only conscious, volitional decision is to reach for the object. The remaining details of the motor event are preprogrammed.

Many learned responses are reflexive and many are preprogrammed in areas [called central pattern generators (CPGs)]. However, motor actions are normally very plastic and adaptable to change. If, for example, the object we are reaching for suddenly moves, we "automatically" and smoothly readjust our movements to the new situation. These automatic readjustments include not only those of the muscles but also the eyes and head, etc.

If trauma compromises the ability to physiologically stimulate more rostral neuraxial centers, the central pattern generators are erroneously programmed resulting in a pathological expression leading to a vicious dysfunctional cycle. Persistent dysfunction stimulates inappropriate plasticity with the ultimate expression of compromise—the inability to make quick and appropriate adjustments to an environmental stimulus. This is an excellent example of dysfunctional display. The erroneous foundation becomes the new "normal" foundation for the more mature neurological display. And that display becomes dysfunctional too, because it is founded on a shaky center.

Dysfunctional Cerebellar Display

Cerebellar motor disturbances express themselves in various ways and can be grouped into nine general categories. Depending on the extent of the cerebellar expression, a person may have one or a combination of these symptoms. In all cases, symptoms from

> Properly integrated postural mechanisms are the motor expression of appropriately organized and adequately facilitated rostral centers.

unilateral cerebellar damage appear on the side ipsilateral to the damage. Ascending spinocerebellar pathways are uncrossed, and descending corticopontocerebellar fibers are crossed. Thus, motor deficits from cerebellar damage are ipsilateral to the lesion, whereas motor deficits from damage to motor areas of the cerebral cortex are contralateral to the lesion.

Table 24: PATHOLOGICAL CEREBELLAR EXPRESSION	
Damage	*Neurological Expression*
Unilateral	Ipsilateral
Motor (Cerebellum)	Ipsilateral
Motor (Cerebral)	Contralateral

The nine categories of pathological cerebellar expression should be examined during every office visit (Table 24). They are:

1) Ataxia: Postural instability—Classified as "-taxias"; involves the limbs, particularly the distal extremities, and is associated with deviations of gait and stance toward the side of the lesion; static and/or dynamic; indicate damage to the vestibulocerebellum

2) Dysmetria: Inability to gauge distance correctly, resulting in premature arrest of movement or overshooting; past pointing or hypermetria; Delayed initiation and termination of motor actions; both are problems when the damage is to the cerebrocerebellum; indicates a lack of coordination of antagonistic muscles and inability to terminate a motor action.

3) Dysdiadochokinesis: Classified as "-kinesias"; inability to perform continuous, repetitive movements; a malfunction of alternating movement; dysrhythmokinesis—an inability to maintain a rhythmic pattern or alternating movements.

4) Intention tremor: Errors in the smoothness and direction of a movement; the movement oscillations become increasingly large as the finger nears the target, producing a kinetic tremor (intention tremor).

5) Asynergia: Loss of coordination or synergy of movement, especially complex movement; most apparent during complex movements; represents a lack of synergy and may take on a step-like pattern; decomposition of movement.

6) Hypotonia: Lack of motor plasticity or motor learning; possible damage to either the inferior olivary nuclei or their projections

fibers, but could be from brain stem damage and not from the cerebellum itself.

7) Rebound phenomenon: caused by an inability to adjust promptly to changes in muscle tension. For example, a person's arm pressed against the hand of the examiner cannot immediately relax when the examiner withdraws his hand but follows the hand with an uncontrolled hitting motion.

8) Scanning speech: asynergia of the muscles of speech results in slow, hesitant, and poorly articulated speech with inappropriate emphasis on individual syllables that cause some words to be uttered explosively.

9) Inability to discriminate weight: an object whose weight is being judged is always believed to be lighter when held in the hand ipsilateral to the cerebellar lesion. This phenomenon is probably related to ipsilateral hypotonia and asthenia.

Recognizing cerebellar display is essential in proper interpretation of functional neurological expression. The more familiar normal is the more obvious pathology appears.

Understanding the normal character of cerebellar display helps realize that which is pathological. This can be done easily with practice and study. Once the dysfunction is isolated, treatment can be directed toward the area causing the dysfunction. This makes the treatment essentially part of the diagnosis because appropriate treatment should not only alleviate the symptoms but also not produce peripheral stress. If peripheral stress does appear, the diagnosis and/or treatment require revision.

Part 7:
Application of Surround Inhibition

Besides the myriad of signals that the entire nervous system must deal with, a healthy cerebellum must maintain an internal organization that will coordinate all the information from both internal and external sources. Further, it must possess properly organized efferent pathways that will allow it to exert its influence upon the segmental apparatus and lower motor centers.

...no matter what nerves go where, the effects of dysfunctional joint motion allow the expression of what should otherwise be inhibited.

When the cumulative effect of peripheral input from joint mechanical receptors together with the right timing increases the membrane potential toward threshold, an action potential is sent along its journey. The part that reaches the cerebellum is finely integrated within its synaptic network and a response is generated. Around 90% of that response will appear in the autonomic centers and only 10% in the muscles. This has profound effects when it comes to treating people properly.

Generally, although a person may have symptoms below the level of T6, the more rostral centers influence what happens in the more caudal centers. That is, the neck generally controls the activities of the lower back and legs, and so forth.

Properly integrated postural mechanisms are the motor expression of appropriately organized and adequately facilitated rostral centers. Further, the functional coordination of autonomic display results in adequately nourished tissues and enhanced functional performance with an absence of pain.

Properly integrated postural mechanisms are the motor expression of appropriately organized and adequately facilitated rostral centers.

Probably the most important cerebellar afferents for upright posture arise from those segments above the level of T6. Earlier, we made reference to the DSCT and CCT tracts. Both traverse the inferior cerebellar peduncle en route to the cerebellum, and both arise generally above T6, having components from both the forelimb and hind limb, but the primary input to the CCT is from the cuneate tract and accessory cuneate nucleus in the medulla, as opposed to the DSCT, which receives input primarily from Clarke's column in the spinal cord.

Since the more rostral centers have a greater neurological influence than those from more caudal areas, upper body exercise has a greater degree of influence over more caudal neurologic display than exercise of more caudal areas.

Most people do lower body cardiovascular exercises like the stationary bicycle, Stairmaster™ and treadmill. While these are good exercises, they each focus on the muscles of the lower extremities in an effort to exercise the heart by bringing blood from the furthest distance. Done inappropriately, they can lead to neurologic compromise and the breakdown of shunt stability with anaerobic function of paraspinal muscles and the consequential biochemical byproducts of joint breakdown by exceeding the functional capacity of the muscles to maintain their endurance nature.

A better way to exercise the heart and the cardiovascular system both aerobically and neurologically is through the upper extremities. Exercising the upper extremities in a functional fashion enhances not only the shunt stability of the intrinsic muscles of the spine and resulting support of cerebellar controls over vital centers, but it also leads to an increased cardiovascular performance with enhanced autonomic controls.

The outflow of both the DSCT and CCT input is through corticonuclear pathways that receive input from Purkinje projections of inhibition resulting from stimulation of basket and stellate cells through the

...anaerobic function is synonymous with short bursts of activity; the adaptation of the paraspinal muscles to this behavior compromises their endurance or shunt character.

mossy and climbing fiber input resulting from primary afferents of joint mechanoreceptor stimulation. The whole design of surround inhibition is to facilitate Purkinje inhibition of the postsynaptic centers, allowing functional integrity of the intrinsic paraspinal muscles for functional motion and to enhance autonomic performance.

Further, since anaerobic function is synonymous with short bursts of activity, the adaptation of the paraspinal muscles to this behavior compromises their endurance or shunt character. They become unable to endure the requirements of stabilization. Then, when the more axial and foundational joints try to support the more peripheral spurt motion, the unsupported foundation moves pathologically, leading to axial skeletal pathology and the production of biochemical agents of structural failure (for example, polyanionic glycosaminoglycans). They stimulate nociceptive receptors that lead to the perception of pain if they are not presynaptically inhibited in the dorsal aspect of the cord. That presynaptic inhibition comes from the large diameter axons from joint mechanoreceptors. If the joints move pathologically, then the presynaptic inhibition cannot occur, and you obtain the display that should have been inhibited—i.e., pain.

> We all have the same neurological anatomy, but we each use our nervous systems differently.

As we discussed, there are three aspects of structural control. They are posture and balance through the axial skeleton providing for tonus of the extremities, control of posture and gait through the function of the trunk and girdles, and axial control and coordination of skilled learned activity. The function of each is dependent on the quality of input received from the periphery and the resulting display of the CIS of the neuraxis.

> A better way to exercise the heart and the cardiovascular system both aerobically and neurologically is through the upper extremities.

We all have the same neurological anatomy, but we display it differently. That is one of the components that make us unique from all other beings. However, no matter what nerves go where, the effects of dysfunctional joint motion allow the expression of what should otherwise be inhibited. As a result, functional display becomes vulnerable due to errors of modulation. The organized motor patterns that were preprogrammed and others that were learned become sacrificed and replaced by a dysfunctional display and its encouraged plasticity, leading to adaptation, compartmentalization and ultimate pathology.

CASE STUDY: Thomas, 42

Brief History

Thomas presented with chronic complaints with his middle back, upper left shoulder blade and soreness in the anterior aspect of his left shoulder with associated weakness. Thomas liked playing basketball, lifting weights and water skiing. He does not recall how he originally hurt his shoulder, and he had the troubles about a year before the problem was found by exploratory arthroscopy.

An MRI of Thomas' left shoulder was negative in anticipation of surgery to repair a "slap lesion" of the biceps, tendon. He had the chronic left shoulder symptoms for quite some time after that. He was treated with physical therapy and epidural cortisone injections to his shoulder and lower cervical spine. He said "it went real bad" after the doctors punctured his dura. The therapy went on for about a year without benefit.

Immediately after the epidural injection, he experienced "huge pressure through the back of my neck". He got a blood patch and was told to lie down for the next seven to eight weeks. About four weeks into his treatment for the puncture, he started to experience headaches in any posture, and he was treated with antibiotics.

At the time of his physical examination with me, Thomas' worst pain was in his head. He described it as "my head is not right on my neck." His pain went through both temples, and pain and tenderness through his occiput, with that of the left side being greater than that of the right. His symptoms become worse the longer he remains upright.

He characterizes his current headache symptoms as "an achy, bony headache and my neck cracks a lot." He started feeling better about eight days before his exam here in my office. He is able to be up for a while without getting into terrible pain. He feels better just after getting up in the morning, but his symptoms increase the more he is upright.

Thomas had a history of a bad auto accident about 13 years earlier. His car was hit from behind and thrown across an island, and then it was hit by another car coming from the other direction. He felt sore for three months after that, but after that he said he felt "fine."

Thomas seems to have lots of cracking and popping in his neck, but never had the same head and neck problems before his epidural.

He feels weak from bed rest and he lost about 36 pounds over the last three to four months.

Further, when he was 14 years old, he was hit in the head by a hardball in little league, and knocked unconscious. He was in intensive care overnight, but released after that. He said he apparently never had any residual problems from it.

Thomas' last treatment was about eight weeks before coming to see me.

Pertinent Examination Findings

During the initial examination, Thomas was found to have a heart rate of 78 beats per minute and his respiratory rate was 18 breaths per minute. His vibratory, pinwheel and light touch senses were all decreased on his right side, and he demonstrated palatal and facial paresis on the left and an inhibition of his left finger extensors and abductors.

The range of motion of the dorsal aspect of his left ribs was limited through $-\theta X$ axial rotation and the range of motion of C4-7 appeared to be limited through $+\theta Z$ axial rotation with a simultaneous $+\theta Y$ axial torque. Prior to treatment, the right blind spot was found to be larger than that of the left.

Manual muscle testing indicated that the psoas major, gluteus medius, straight head of the rectus femoris, sartorius and hamstrings were all unable to meet the demands of manual muscle testing, bilaterally. The bilaterally functionally inhibited psoas major remained functionally inhibited when the patient turned his head contralaterally. The bilaterally functionally inhibited gluteus medius remained functionally inhibited when the patient turned his head ipsilaterally. The bilaterally functionally inhibited straight head of the rectus femoris remained functionally inhibited after tapping the deep tendon reflex at the insertion, ipsilaterally. The bilaterally functionally inhibited hamstrings remained functionally inhibited after tapping the deep tendon reflex of the insertions, both medially and laterally, and at the origin. Stroking the sole of the patient's foot with a sharp object displayed a dysfunctional flexor withdrawal response, bilaterally.

Clinical Assessment

This patient appears to be experiencing an increased aspect of left hemisphericity with a concomitant left pyramidal distribution of weakness with autonomic concomitants as a result of a deafferentation of the zygapophyseal joint mechanoreceptors.

Discussion

Thomas is demonstrating a pyramidal distribution of weakness and many autonomic concomitants as a manifestation of a deafferentation of his paraspinal series elastic elements, which have sacrificed their shunt stability in favor of more spurt-like motion.

Further, there appears to be a breakdown of the tonic neck and tonic labyrinthine reflexes, the deep tendon reflexes and flexor withdrawal response, bilaterally. This leads to the inability of the more rostral neurological centers to functionally support the reflexes and therefore the joint stability of the lower extremities.

As a result, the spinal structures appear to be unable to endure as they should leading to a reduction in their ability to adequately afferentate the more rostral neuraxial centers with the production of biochemical end-products that conflict with normal local metabolic pathways. This allows the inability to properly modulate the dorsal aspect of the cord with resulting conscious recognition of nociceptive reflexogenic afferents as well as dysmodulation of the vital centers of the midbrain allowing the expression of that which should be inhibited.

Treatment

Besides supporting the paraspinal structures with physical therapy procedures and rehabilitation exercises consistent with his left pyramidal distribution of weakness, the patient was adjusted with coupled manual manipulative reductive techniques directed toward those joints demonstrating a resistance to motion. He was also given certain specific nutritional supplements to support the biochemical pathways necessary for his heeling.

Prognosis

The prognosis for this patient's recovery is generally good. Following treatment, there was a tremendous improvement in the physical examination and manual muscle testing findings, bilaterally. Together, these positive changes indicated the accuracy of the diagnosis and the appropriateness of care described above.

Part 8:
Summary of Surround Inhibition

Surround inhibition is one of the most important neurological expressions of the human nervous system—the ability to stand upright and support the metabolic demands of that effort.

Understanding the processes of surround inhibition can be very complex. Yet, once you understand the processes of neurological display they become clearer. The key is to appreciate the neurological pathways and their function. With that, the intricacies are more familiar and comfortable.

Motor tasks are both preprogrammed and learned. The former are preset in central areas that generate the coordination of body patterns (central pattern generators CPG's). The latter are developed through their involvement in planning and initiation of skilled movement.

However, motor actions are normally very plastic and adaptable to change. Reflexes like the tonic neck, tonic labyrinthine, deep tendon and crossed extensor together with the flexor reflex afferents display relative to the integrity of their homologous columns. If the pathways of performance are physiologically stimulated, the motor response will be likewise physiological. But if they are dysfunctionally stimulated as a result of improper function, the resultant display will also be dysfunctional. Since dysfunction is synonymous with pathology, the display represents functional illness not only in the structure but also in the autonomic concomitants consistent with that display.

Appropriate treatment is essential for reduction of the pathological display, otherwise peripheral stress appears leading to further adaptation and pathology.

Pathological motion leads to the inability to knock out nociception in the dorsal aspects of the spinal cord, and the conscious recognition of that stimulus we know to be pain. It also generates dysfunctional modulation of that part of the spinal cord that controls autonomic function allowing the expression of autonomic display that should have otherwise been eliminated.

Examining Multiarticulate Muscles

Analyzing Their Role in Functional Joint Integrity

Introduction

Of the over 600 muscles that provide human locomotion, the great majority of them are uniarticulate (Figure 85), i.e., they cross only one joint but move two bones.

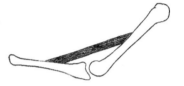

Figure 85: A uniarticulate muscle crosses one joint but moves two bones

Several biarticulate (Figure 86) muscles cross two joints and move three bones.

Triarticulate muscles (Figure 87) are the smallest and most unique of the multiarticulate muscles. Multiarticulate muscles act in unusual ways, sometimes having different actions at their ends and at other times working each end together for one uniform act. They contract less but generate greater movement; an energy conservation technique. That makes their examination unique and their treatment fundamental to the fixed action patterns (FAPs) characteristic of the preprogrammed human design.

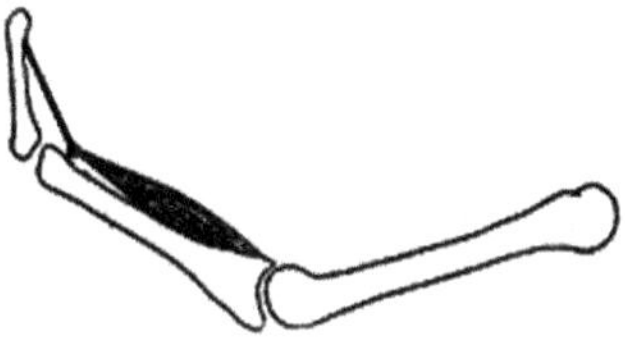

Figure 86: An example of a biarticulate (flexor) muscle of the finger, which affects two joints and three bones

Functional Neurology

It appears that the past two decades have seen a revival in the application of manual muscle testing as functional neurology (fMMT). The work of George Goodheart, DC—the founder of applied

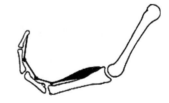

Figure 87: An example of a triarticulate (flexor) muscle of the finger, which affects three joints and four bones

kinesiology— and the application of functional neurological principles taught by Carrick have shed new light and given greater understanding of the concepts of using manual muscle testing as functional neurology.

There is definitely a hierarchical arrangement to the functional human nervous system, and when that inborn order breaks down, so do the controls that make it uniquely human. This breakdown consists of timing errors, deafferentation, inflammatory responses and atypical joint reciprocity resulting in a decreased potentiation of normal reciprocal movement that impairs cognitive abilities. In the wake of this breakdown is joint stress, an increased potential for injury, and pain.

Discussion

The standard anatomical philosophy of how certain muscle groups control isolated joint flexion, extension and rotation, identifies which muscles should be trained to enhance sports performance. But what if that muscle's apparent need for training is the result of atypical feedback from the CNS instead of the actual need to work harder? The movement that is on display, rather than being consistent with the original human programming, may be totally "sub-human" with erroneous patterns of facilitation and inhibition.

It may seem right to exercising a conditionally inhibited muscle to make it stronger but it could be exactly the wrong thing to do relative to the CIS of the anterior horn of the spinal cord if the muscle's controls are inconsistent with its original programming.

Two Examples of fMMT

The typical start position for a manual muscle test (MMT) that isolates its involved joint(s) as used by applied kinesiologists is usually done as if the muscle spans only one joint. The muscle test (Table 25) is readied

Table 25:
Muscles Displayed in this Chapter

- Pectoralis major, clavicular portion (Figure 88)
- Rectus femoris (Figures 93 and 94)
- Quadriceps (Figure 95)
- Hamstrings (Figures 89 and 90)
- Biceps brachii (Figure 91)
- Brachialis (Figure 92)

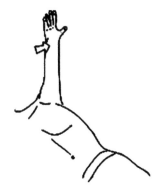

Figure 88: The start position to test the clavicular portion of the pectoralis major (PMC)

by moving the bones that incorporate the origin and insertion of the muscle closer together and testing the muscle by pushing to separate them. The start position to test the clavicular portion of the pectoralis major PMC (Figure 88) is an excellent example. It takes its origin from the medial third of the clavicle and inserts into the intertubercular groove or outer lip of the proximal anterior humerus.The examiner asks the patient to raise their upper extremity so that the shoulder is flexed to 90°, with the elbow straight and the arm is rotated inward (this can be done in any posture, standing, sitting, or supine). The practitioner stands to the side of the patient, supports the near shoulder with the nearest hand, and checks the integrity of the muscle with the other hand contacting the patient's forearm just proximal to the wrist joint. The test pressure is in the direction that follows the line of the muscle fibers—abduction with very slight extension.

As with most other muscles, the PMC can be tested with both eccentric and concentric testing. These tests—and when necessary their treatment—can bring clinical benefit to the patient. The problem is that not all muscles are simply uniarticulate.

The standard prone group hamstrings test is another good example. The group hamstring test is often performed as if it were a uniarticulate muscle when, in fact, only the short head of the biceps femoris (Figure 91) is uniarticulate. While the semimembranosus, semitendinosus and biceps femoris all arise from a common origin their insertions are unique. Aside from the short head of the biceps femoris, the hamstring's course crosses two joints making them biarticulate.

When we understand the dynamics of afferents from each of these muscles to the spinal cord and the motor responses that result these afferents, we can recognize even greater clinical significance to these tests and their ultimate effect on the more rostral neuraxis.

Uniarticulate Muscles

This paper suggests a modification of the standard muscle testing strategies that accompanies the usual isolated joint test. There must be an awareness of the anatomical arrangement of muscles relative to their involved joints and how each muscle contributes to that joint's movement.

The motion of one segment affects the motions at all segments to which the first segment is linked. This is the idea of homologous columns and relates to issues of joint stability. A joint's stability is relative to the preprogrammed inhibitory cascade that flows from the rostral neuraxis. This cascade can affect joint movement both favorably and unfavorably—both functionally and dysfunctionally. Whenever a body segment is moved, muscles acting on homologous segments must be activated to produce shunt stability that prevents undesired movement. However, when the movements are inconsistent with those that are preprogrammed into the human neurological matrix or their signals are mismatched due to deafferentation conditions, the result is a functional instability that affects more peripheral movements. Hence afferent latency is particularly important.

A muscle's dysfunction should not be interpreted only in terms of its action at the joint or joints that it spans, but also upon those muscles far afield from the lesion that might be produced by a dysfunction. An important natural action of a muscle's function may be to produce motion at a remote joint by means of reaction torques. The tonic neck reflex (TNR), tonic labyrinthine reflex (TLR), flexor reflex afferent (FRA), crossed cord reflex (CCR), and deep tendon reflex (DTR), etc., are excellent examples of the aspects of the functional matrix that help muscles maintain homologous integrity, but also can be reasons for erroneous performance when the preprogrammed patterns of any one or a combination of these reflexes becomes compromised. Each of these reflexes has an accompanying postural display relative to its distance from the original stimulus. They have their individual effects but they work together as a functional unit that yields natural human movement patterns. As a result, a small motion at a proximal joint can be transformed into a much larger expression at a distal joint. However, if a muscle is unable to endure through its entire range of functional abilities its requisite factors will compromise the performance of more remote areas dependent upon the dysfunctional muscle, resulting in structural breakdown.

The mechanical impediment of a limb's functional movement plays an important role in the breakdown of not only its afferents but also to its global postural stability. Any hindrance of the foundational muscles (i.e., shunt stabilizers) that steady the skeleton in advance of a voluntary perturbing action of a limb's movement can be dangerous. This signal is modulated via the basal ganglia, cerebellum and cortex, as well as the intervening control centers that make up the central pattern generators (CPG) or pre-programmed movement patterns, but if these controlling factors are themselves compromised then the structure submissive to them will be likewise compromised.

Biarticulate Muscles

While uniarticulate muscles appear to be activated for movements in a preferred direction that may be correlated to the direction of maximum shortening regardless of direction of externally applied force. Biarticulate muscles have a more complicated display. This is the general idea of fMMT and multiarticulate muscles; isolate that aspect of a muscle in question in its maximum contraction and push against it. The old ideas of manual muscle testing must be advanced because there is so much more to be observed and learned. It is time to go to the next level of manual muscle testing: fMMTs.

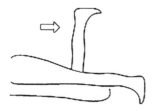

Figure 89: The standard prone position to test the distal portion of the hamstrings as a group

It is not a straightforward matter to predict the activation pattern of a set of muscles when these biarticulate muscles act on multiple limb segments or about multiple axes of rotation. But we have an advantage with fMMT. Whether a muscle acts as an agonist, antagonist or stabilizer will depend on factors such as joint angles, link lengths, moment arms, and force directions. However, the most important factor in the consideration of limb movement is the CIS of the anterior horn of the spinal cord because it is the final common pathway and it is influenced by so many factors.Biarticulate muscles appear to be used to control force direction regardless of whether they shorten or lengthen. Biarticulate

245

muscles can serve to reduce the amount of work that muscles must absorb (negative work) when a joint must rotate in one direction, but generate torque in the opposite direction. This happens frequently when the direction of force at the endpoint of the limb must be controlled.

Hamstrings

The hamstrings are another muscle commonly used for fMMT. There are a variety of ways to test the hamstrings [i.e., lying prone (Figure 89) or supine (Figure 90), sitting, or standing] and all are appropriate but they yield different information. The muscle is most commonly

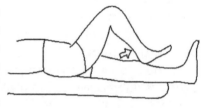

Figure 90: Supine hamstring test

tested with the patient prone, but it can also be tested in the supine posture; the leg is flexed on the thigh in the former, but while the same is true in the latter the thigh is also flexed on the hip.

Biceps brachii and brachialis

In many cases, one muscle will couple a joint's torque about two axes of rotation, such as the biceps brachii (Figure 91), which couples

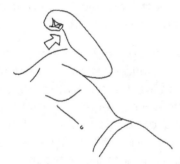

Figure 91: The position to test the
short head of the biceps brachii

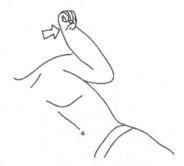

Figure 92: The position
to test the brachialis

elbow flexion and supination. In certain conditions, this coupling can produce undesired torque problems with pain and joint breakdown that must be counterbalanced by other muscles. Similarly, shoulder muscles may contribute to force in both desired and undesired directions at the hand. Again, these undesired forces must be counterbalanced by the actions of muscles that produce forces in opposite directions. How else can the doctor know the functional stability of these muscles if he or she does not test them against themselves and other muscles?

Quadriceps

Another common example is the quadriceps. While the vastus muscles are uniarticulate, the rectus femoris muscle (Figures 93 and 94) is biarticulate; in fact it has a straight head (Figure 95) and a reflected head (not shown).

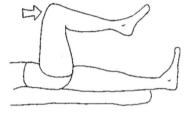

Figure 93: The start position to test the proximal rectus femoris

The quadriceps group is often tested in the supine posture with the thigh flexed on the hip and the leg flexed on the thigh, with pressure applied at the distal thigh as if to extend the thigh on the hip (Figure 93), but this test isolates the proximal rectus femoris. Another version of this muscle test is to have the patient in the same posture but applying pressure to the ankle as if to flex the knee further (Figure 94).

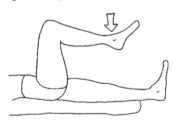

Figure 94: The start position to test the distal rectus femoris

Each of these quadriceps muscle test is a valuable part of our fMMT armamentarium because each one tests something different. The first test focuses more on the origin of the rectus femoris while the second test involves a group quadriceps test (the vastus muscles and the rectus femoris) since they have a common insertion (Figure 95). The key to each muscle's function lies in the central integrative state of the anterior horn of the spinal cord—the final common pathway—at the level of the test, in these cases the spinal cord segments are L2-4. In order to appreciate a somatic awareness of the afferent signals from the proximal aspect of the rectus femoris relative to its distal aspect, the segmental cohesion of the cord must be oriented rostrocaudally. Further, the proximal aspect relatively isolates the muscle's origin while the distal aspect of the rectus femoris test gathers involvement of the vastus muscles.

These concepts are important when dealing with the subsequent discussion of multiarticulate muscles below.

Multiarticulate Muscles

Many muscles—or their tendons—span more than one joint (Table 26). Biarticulate muscles are the most common of the multiarticulate type while the tendon of insertion of some finger flexors and extensors cross up to four joints.

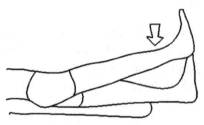

Figure 95: The start position to test the straight head of the rectus femoris (the quadriceps group)

The existence of muscles that span several joints can provide a number of advantages of the musculoskeletal system. In the case of the fingers and wrist, most of the muscle mass is removed from the hand, reducing the inertia and allowing rapid response.

All motor signals cascade to the anterior horn of the spinal cord. Whether or not higher centers enter into the activities of the cord or if a reflex action is working independently as a fixed action pattern, the CIS of the anterior horn is influenced by the sum total of all inhibitory postsynaptic potentials (IPSPs) and excitatory postsynaptic potentials (EPSPs) affecting that segment, i.e., segmental CIS.

Most muscles require the reciprocal coordination of all the involved muscles acting at several joints. Some muscles act as movers, some as stabilizers and others as breaks. The breaking signal is as important as the motor signal because it helps generate tone and cord modulation. Unlike single joint movements where only the muscles attached to a limb segment can accelerate or decelerate it, in multi-joint movements, distant muscles can perform the same actions.

The dynamics of limb movement dictate that the angular acceleration at any joint is affected by the torques produced at all of the other limb joints. This means, for example, that acceleration of the shoulder is affected by torque at the elbow and vice versa. Thus, muscles that cross only the elbow joint can influence the angular acceleration of the shoulder.

Since muscles can act as agonists, synergists or antagonists in different situations, the pattern of activation depends on the direction of motion, which is modulated at the anterior horn of the cord. If a joint's function is aberrant, its deafferentation results in movement error. Consequently, different muscles will be activated at unusual latencies with respect to movement onset with the possibility of resulting problems. Similarly, a given muscle can be activated at latencies that are outside normal limits depending on the movement direction. Because aberrant joint motion produces deafferentation, a proprioceptive breakdown can lead to the dysmodulation of nociception in the dorsal horn of the spinal cord and the eventual realization of pain.

Synergistic Movement

Frequently, the motion at neighboring joints is such that biarticulate muscles undergo smaller changes in length than uniarticulate muscles. Consequently, the muscle fibers do not undergo large changes in length and can remain on a favorable region of their length-tension curve. They will also have smaller shortening velocities, allowing them to produce higher forces during contraction. For example, during locomotion, the knee and ankle often flex and extend together, minimizing the length change that occurs in the gastrocnemius muscle.

Among the issues influencing segmental cord modulation are movement velocities and joint stabilities of all those signals that have influence on that segment or those segments involved. Even a joint far removed from that in question can have influence on segmental performance through its modulatory influences. That type of cooperative interaction between the muscle groups is what results in functional, sequential muscle actions and skilled movement. There must be teamwork between the muscles most involved and their contralateral (agonists, antagonists, and synergists, both ipsilateral and contralateral) or reciprocal muscles. The actions of reciprocally working muscles often vary depending upon the skills being performed. For example, the hamstrings and quadriceps must work reciprocally when walking, running or riding a bicycle. This is synergistic movement.

A biarticulate muscle that crosses two joints influences three bones and has parallel axes of rotation that can either accelerate both joints in the same direction as the direction of the torque, which it produces, or it can accelerate one of the joints in the direction opposite to the direction of the torque that it produces at the joint.

Table 26: EXAMPLES OF MULTIARTICULATE MUSCLES	
Biarticulate muscles (span two joints)	**Multiarticulate muscles (span three or four joints; found in the most distal joints of the fingers and toes**
Biceps brachii	Extensor carpi radialis longus
Triceps brachii	Extensor carpi radialis brevis
Sartorius	Extensor carpi ulnaris
Rectus femoris	Extensor indicus
Semitendinosus	Extensor digiti minimi
Semimembranosus	Extensor pollicus longus
Biceps femoris (long head)	Extensor pollicus brevis
Gastrocnemius	Extensor digitorum
	Extensor digiti minimi
	Flexor digitorum profundus
	Flexor carpi ulnaris
	Flexor carpi radialis
	Flexor digitorum superficialis
	Flexor pollicus longus
	Palmaris longus

The gastrocnemius muscle is a biarticulate muscle that produces an extensor torque at the ankle and a flexor torque at the knee. Its action at the two joints is determined by the ratio of its moment arms at the knee and ankle and by the knee angle. The gastrocnemius could 1) flex the knee and extend the ankle, 2) extend the knee and extend the ankle, or 3) flex the knee and flex the ankle. These effects are the result of the combined direct action of the muscle at the joint and the indirect effect of the reaction torque at the knee produced by the acceleration of the shank at the ankle.

Another example is the rectus femoris muscle. When the proximal rectus femoris contracts fully, the thigh flexes on the pelvis and the leg extends on the thigh. At the same instant, the proximal and distal aspects of the hamstrings must relax allowing the femur to move forward in the swing phase of gait. Just before the heel strikes the ground, the distal rectus femoris must relax so that the knee can flex. That flexion is associated with facilitation of the distal hamstrings. The transition phase sees the facilitation of the distal rectus femoris with the inhibition of the distal hamstrings while the proximal rectus femoris inhibits with the facilitation of the proximal hamstrings. There are many other signals being transmitted simultaneously, but these are just a few in order to help make the point of synergistic movement. Muscles must work reciprocally, and their modulation is segmental relative to the CIS of the anterior horn.

Multiarticulate muscles generate unique aspects of joint stability and movement not seen in uniarticulate muscles. By virtue of their structure, they conserve energy and enhance joint stability. Their afferentation demands complex response patterns depending upon their latency, causing certain aspects of joint motion locally and structural integrity distally.

Movement of the hand or fingertip often follows a path that is almost straight. This requires the coordinated action of several joints moving in parallel at different angular velocities and sometimes in different directions. Angular acceleration or angular velocity at one joint may create an undesired torque at another joint due to reaction forces or motion dependent forces such as centrifugal and Coriolus effects. Joint stiffness will help to limit the perturbing effect of torque; the stiffer the joint, the less the undesired movement. Although such motion dependent torques will increase with movement speed, muscle activation will also increase, resulting in increased joint stiffness, which may help to offset the effects of greater perturbing torques.

Primitive Reflex Involvement

The Normal Deep Tendon Reflex (DTR)

When the origin or insertion of a muscle is struck briskly, the stimulus should cause the functional facilitation of the stimulated muscle for one muscle test with the functional inhibition of its antagonist(s).

The Normal Asymmetrical Tonic Neck Reflex (ATNR)

In general, turning the head to one side should cause the functional facilitation of the extensors, external rotators and abductors on the side toward head rotation, and a functional inhibition of the flexors, internal rotators and adductors ipsilaterally. Further, there should be a concomitant functional facilitation of the flexors, internal rotators and adductors on the side opposite head rotation, and a concomitant functional inhibition of the extensors, external rotators and abductors ipsilaterally. This is true for both the upper and lower extremities.

The Normal Symmetrical Tonic Neck Reflex (ATNR)

A flexion synergy functionally facilitates the upper extremity flexors and lower extremity extensors while an extension synergy functionally facilitates the upper extremity extensors and lower extremity flexors.

The Normal Tonic Labyrinthine Reflex (TLR)

With the patient in the supine posture, there should be a generalized functionally facilitation of the muscles of extension while the muscles of flexion should be generally functionally facilitated in the prone patient.

The Normal Crossed Cord Reflex (CCR) Response

There are any combination of 12 different cord-centered events subsequent to a primary afferent stimulus (from somatic tissue such as muscles, joints and skin) reaching the cord. Eight of these twelve responses have to do with upper and lower extremity posture. Any response other than that which is anticipated should always be considered to be pathological; "sub-human."

The Normal Flexor Reflex Afferent (FRA) Response

This reflex is normally protective. Stroking the sole of the foot with a sharp object should cause the functional facilitation of physiological flexors and functional inhibition of physiological extensors of the lower extremity ipsilateral to the stimulus with a concomitant functional inhibition of the physiological flexors and functional facilitation of the physiological extensors of the lower extremity contralateral to the stimulus. Moreover, there should also be a functional facilitation of the physiological flexors and functional inhibition of the physiological extensors of the upper extremity contralaterally and a functional facilitation of the physiological extensors and functional inhibition of the physiological flexors of the upper extremity ipsilaterally.

A special note: because of the construction of this FRA reflex—its protective nature—the stroking stimulus and its resultant postural response decays over a three to five second period. Further, the stimulation of this reflex takes precedence over any other such stimulus, i.e., a second FRA stimulus overrides a previous FRA stimulus, which causes the latter to display subsequent to the former.

The Normal Galant Reflex Response (GR)

Stroking the lumbar flank (below T6) with a sharp object rostrocaudally causes a functional facilitation of the hip flexors and adductors with a functional inhibition of the knee extensors and abductors ipsilaterally. Concomitantly, there should be a functional inhibition of the hip extensors and abductors ipsilaterally with an associated functional facilitation of the hip extensors and abductors contralaterally.

The Normal Modified Galant Reflex Response (MGR)

Stroking the thoracic spine (above T6) about one to two inches lateral to its spinous processes rostrocaudally causes a functional facilitation of the hamstrings group test ipsilaterally while tapping the same area of the dorsal spine causes a functional inhibition of the hamstrings ipsilaterally.

The Upper Galant Reflex Response (UGR)

Stroking the thoracic spine (above T6) about one to two inches lateral to its spinous processes rostrocaudally causes a functional inhibition of the ipsilateral deltoid and a functional facilitation of the ipsilateral PMC. Conversely, tapping the same areas of the upper dorsal spine (above T6) with a sharp object rostrocaudally causes a functional inhibition of the PMC and a functional facilitation of the deltoid ipsilaterally.

Combining Various Stimuli

Dealing with multiarticulate muscles requires the examiner to work "outside the box." Any muscle will respond to reflexive testing and the information obtained is quite beneficial to the treatment of the case. The consideration is whether the observed response is consistent with that which would be anticipated. If it is, then the system is normal, but if not then there is pathology within the sensory and/or motor display.

There are several aspects of muscle function to consider, to examine, and to reexamine during each patient's treatment. For example, the doctor must compare the PMC not only to the various primitive reflexes related to that muscle's function but also to the different aspects of gait and gravity. The same muscle can—and often will— behave differently relative to the various stimuli placed on it and to simply examine a muscle as if it were a uniarticulate muscle and consider that to be normal is often misleading. The doctor must combine different aspects of each muscle's dynamic and not only to it, but also to any and all other muscles that are homologously related.

Summary

Many muscles have only two attachments—one at each end. However, the more complex muscles are often attached to several different structures at their origins and/or their insertion, i.e., the biceps brachii, the triceps brachii, and the quadriceps. If these attachments are separated, effectively meaning that the muscle gives rise to two or more tendons and/or *aponeuroses* inserting into different places, then the muscle is said to have two heads. The biceps brachii has two heads at its origin: one from the coracoid process and other from the supraglenoid tubercle. Similarly, the triceps has three heads and the quadriceps have four.

All aspects of a muscle's performance must be taken into consideration when testing these muscles. Further, there are aspects of neurological performance that also come into play with muscle stability and performance. Each of these aspects has its influence on the cord and more rostral neuraxis.

Case Study #12

History and Presenting Complaints: Eileen, 16; loves to play water polo. She complained of pain on the inside of her left knee with every kick as she circumducts her left leg medially while treading water.

Exam Findings: During the course of a normal physical examination it was observed that the following muscles appeared to be unable to meet the demands of manual muscle testing, bilaterally: rectus femoris, psoas major, sartorius, gluteus medius, tensor fascia lata, hamstrings, piriformis, and popliteus, all of which involve her knees.

The rectus femoris appeared to be functionally inhibited bilaterally without functional facilitation upon tapping the distal aspect of the rectus femoris ipsilaterally. Further, the rectus femoris appeared to be functionally inhibited bilaterally with functional facilitation upon tapping the origin of the rectus femoris, ipsilaterally.

The psoas major appeared to be functionally inhibited without facilitation with the patient's head rotated contralaterally, but with facilitation with the patient's head rotated ipsilaterally. The sartorius appeared to be functionally inhibited bilaterally without functional facilitation with the patient's head rotated contralaterally. The gluteus medius appeared to be functionally inhibited bilaterally without functional facilitation with the patient's head rotated ipsilaterally, but with facilitation with the patient's head rotated contralaterally. The tensor fascia lata appeared to be functionally inhibited without functional facilitation with the patient's head rotated ipsilaterally, but with facilitation with the patient's head rotated contralaterally. The popliteus appeared to be functionally inhibited without facilitation with the patient's head rotated ipsilaterally.

Stroking the sole of the patient's foot with a sharp object appeared to cause inhibition of the rectus femoris ipsilaterally with a concomitant facilitation of the hamstrings contralaterally.

In the prone posture, the hamstrings appeared to be functionally inhibited bilaterally without functional facilitation upon tapping the deep tendon reflex at its origin and/or insertion ipsilaterally, but with facilitation when stroking the Galant reflex contralaterally. The piriformis appeared to be functionally inhibited bilaterally without functional facilitation with the patient's head rotated ipsilaterally, but with facilitation when stroking the Galant reflex ipsilaterally.

Clinical Impression: The patient's functional condition appears to be contrary to structural stability with a demonstrable dysfunction of her reflexive performance.

Treatment Plan: The patient will receive coupled chiropractic manual manipulative procedures to her spine and spinal related structures in order to cure or relieve her condition and reestablish normal neurophysiological responses. She will also receive structural rehabilitation exercises consistent with her treatments.

Response to Care: Immediately after treatment the patient experienced a relief of her knee pain.

Discussion: The patient's pain was the result of her inability to presynaptically inhibit nociceptive reflexogenic afferents in the dorsal aspect of her spinal cord. As a result, she had pain with every knee movement. Reestablishing the normal reciprocal movements necessary for increased joint stability returned the normal and preprogrammed human movement parameters with a concomitant reduction of pain.

A Discussion of the Pyramidal Distribution of Weakness

Gaining a Better Understanding of the Stroke Antalgia Posture

Introduction

This paper deals with the physiological effects of a pyramidal distribution of weakness (PDW) and how to evaluate it with the functional neurological techniques of applied kinesiology. Further, it details certain specific exercise techniques necessary to physiologically facilitate those areas of the neuraxis that have become hyperpolarized, thereby providing for the normalization of the physiological processes that bring the deafferentated areas back to threshold.

The key to understanding the PDW is awareness that the entire human nervous system is receptor based. All aspects of human performance are as a result of the signals that arise from afferent input largely as a result of joint mechanoreceptor function.

We know that differences exist in the delicate membrane potential balance between the internal and external environments of a neuron. These differences can be observed in the laboratory as the resting membrane potential. But as a result of the complexities of human behavior and environmental stimulation, it is doubtful that such a resting state could exist in living tissue. In fact, in man, there is always a constant flux of membrane potential differences that occur as a result of changes in spatial and temporal summation, pH, oxygen tissue saturation and temperature. This constant flux can be clinically seen as shifts toward either depolarization or hyperpolarization, or toward a more or less excited state. The point is that the function of the human nervous system is an integration of all those things that collectively result in potential differences across the neuronal membrane barrier. The integration of these effects is different at individual neurons, and at different times during human performance, due to the interrelationships of all those signals that come from the periphery to the central neuraxis and those that proceed from the central neuraxis to the periphery.

As a result, the description of the differences in membrane potential can be referred to as its CIS. This term has profound clinical ramifications as the clinician can augment a multitude of factors that, in and of themselves, can change the functional state of a neuron and provide far reaching understanding of the nervous system's presentation, and indicate the proper therapeutic response.

An adequate afferent input brings the CIS of the neuraxis to a condition of functional readiness, thereby potentiating the motor response toward sodium equilibrium potential, or threshold. Deafferentation, on the other hand, drives the CIS of the neuraxis toward potassium equilibrium potential, or away from threshold, and results in a degenerative change in the functional status of its postsynaptic tissues that would otherwise affect a task other than the one they are producing as a result of that deafferentation. This allows the compromise that the controlling systems would have prevented, hence the production of the PDW.

Discussion

The Afferent System

The main afferents to the somatosensory centers come from the graded, non-propagated action potentials that arise in the receptors in the organs of balance, the proprioceptors of the neck, and from the cerebellum (tonic labyrinthine and tonic neck reflexes). They are organized in a rostral-caudal fashion, with the highest priority in the upper spine as opposed to the lower spine, the upper extremity as opposed to the lower extremity, and the upper part of the upper extremity as opposed to the lower part of the upper extremity.

Joint mechanoreceptors, particularly those of the axial skeleton, send afferent signals to the spinal cord via type Ia fibers. Their second order neurons terminate in the thalamus and cerebellum. And from the cerebellum, they ultimately reach the thalamus. The point is that all sensory afferents (except those of the sense of smell) ultimately terminate in the thalamus. From there, they project to the cerebrum as third order neurons via the corona radiata.

The somesthetic sensory cortex (areas 3, 1 and 2 of the postcentral gyrus of the frontal lobe) receives afferentation from the periphery in a somatotopically organized fashion such that the upper body components are represented rostral to those of the lower body, and projects its fibers to the motor cortex via engram cells, or cerebral interneuronal projections.

The sum of all the excitatory and inhibitory input to the sensory nervous system determines the CIS of the higher levels of the neuraxis. However, an increased level of excitatory stimulation does not necessarily mean an increased level of overall function if those excitatory stimuli excite inhibitory neurons. This can lead to an increased dampening of function with a decrease in overall excitability. The point is that any deafferentation of these tracts will tend to drive the postsynaptic, neurons more toward potassium equilibrium potential, causing them to be less responsive to their afferent input. This creates a decreased ability to excite the inhibitory neurons, leading to consequential hyperactivity of those areas that would have otherwise been modulated by those inhibitory neurons.

The Efferent System

The motor cortex is divided into two separate divisions, the premotor (areas 4s and 6) and primary (area 4) motor areas. The premotor area lies just anterior to the primary motor area in the precentral gyrus. Very few premotor fibers project directly to the spinal cord via the pyramidal tract. Instead, most of the pyramidal fibers originate in areas 4s and 6, and cause more complex muscle movements, usually involving groups of muscles performing some specific task, rather than to individual muscles.

Pyramidal tract fibers originating in areas 4s and 6 do not initiate impulses to voluntary muscles, but act as inhibitors, suppressors, or "brakes" on the lower motor neurons and prevent them from over discharging when responding reflexively to sensory stimuli. If for some reason motor neurons are freed from their inhibitory or modulatory control, they discharge spontaneously in response to the segmental reflex stimuli to that they are usually dampened. This is due to an inhibition of the inhibitory controls. In other words, the nerves are allowed to do that which they are usually inhibited from doing.

To achieve their results, the premotor area mainly sends its signals into the primary motor cortex to excite multiple groups of muscles. Some of these signals pass directly to the motor cortex through subcortical nerve fibers. But the premotor cortex also has extensive connections with the basal ganglia and cerebellum, both of which transmit signals back by way of the thalamus to the motor cortex. Thus, the premotor cortex, the basal ganglia, the cerebellum, and the primary motor cortex constitute a complex overall system for voluntary control of muscle activity called the corticolenticulopallidostriatothalamocortical feedback loop.

A major share of the output signals from the basal ganglial system is inhibitory. Much of this inhibition feeds back to the primary motor cortex to inhibit the pyramidal system itself, but still additional inhibitory signals pass into the brain stem to inhibit depolarization of the reticular formation and therefore the autonomic fibers, and vestibular nuclei. Therefore, release of these other motor neurons from the basal ganglial inhibition allows for an inhibition of the normal inhibitory function, or an excess excitatory motor response, leading to reflexogenic muscle spasm and autonomic concomitants.

The primary motor cortex receives the bulk of the input from its engram cells, which are postsynaptic to the somatosensory cortex. From here, the primary motor cortex sends its fibers to the spinal cord and brain stem without synapse through the corticospinal (pyramidal) and corticobulbar (extrapyramidal) tracts, respectively.

The pyramidal tract is that neurological tract which has to do with fine voluntary and purposeful motor function. It is universally regarded as the descending pathway most concerned with voluntary, discrete, skilled movements of the distal extremities, it travels caudally to the pyramids of the medulla where approximately 80-90% of the fibers decussate to the contralateral side and become known as the crossed pyramidal or lateral corticospinal tract. The other 10-20% of the fibers remain ipsilateral and descend as the uncrossed (direct) pyramidal tract or anterior corticospinal tract. They terminate by synapsing with motoneurons in the anterior horn of the spinal cord.

The extrapyramidal system is much older than the pyramidal system. Its purpose is twofold. First, it acts to dampen the strong facilitory influence of the pyramidal tract. Second, it modulates the autonomic functions of the intermediolateral cell column, which takes its most rostral origin in the Edinger-Westphal nucleus of the third cranial nerve.

The extrapyramidal tract is also concerned to a great extent with protection. For example, when only the extrapyramidal system is functional, stimuli to the bottom of the feet causes a typical withdrawal protective type of reflex that is expressed by the upturned great toe and fanning of the other toes. But, when the pyramidal system is also fully functional, it suppresses the protective reflex and instead excites a higher order of motor function, including the normal effect of causing downward bending of the toes in response to sensory stimuli from the bottom of the feet. As we shall see, this becomes very important in the diagnosis of the PDW.

Modulation

Specifically, the descending cascade of the extrapyramidal tract synapses in multiple areas: The basal ganglia, thalamus, the subthalamic nucleus of Luys, substantia nigra, red nucleus, reticular formation, pontine nuclei (and therefore cerebellar afferents and efferents through their homologous interneurons), inferior olive and spinal interneurons. The nucleus of Luys and substantia nigra send postsynaptic fibers to the red nucleus and reticular formation both ipsilaterally and contralaterally, while red nucleus and reticular formation send their terminal fibers to the cord. The red nucleus sends its efferents contralaterally to terminate on the ventral horn cells of the spinal cord. The reticular formation sends its efferent fibers to the cord both ipsilaterally and contralaterally. Because these fibers can arise from the thalamus via the hypothalamus without cortical tributaries, this tract is also known as the thalamohypothalamoreticulospinal tract, and its function is modulatory.

Considering the above, we find that the pyramidal and extrapyramidal tracts have almost direct communication with their anterior motoneurons of the cord for control of either individual muscles or small groups of muscles. This may be seen as purposeful motion or postural control, and is distinguished mainly in cervical segments with diminishing influence as it progresses caudally.

Deafferentation of the cerebral cortex can affect not only its somesthetic sense areas but also its motor responses. If that area is not brought: to threshold, it is said to be driven more toward potassium equilibrium potential, adversely effecting its ability to perform its requisite tasks resulting in dysfunction arid the clinical symptoms of stroke antalgia, but without the tissue pathology seen concomitant with a vascular accident.

Not only do the skeletal muscles demonstrate the stroke antalgia in the form of a certain and specific postural gait, but also autonomic concomitants which are the same as, but not as a result of the patient having had a stroke. However, as a result of a hyperpolarization of those pathways that supply the vascular tissues, there can by a change in the blood supply to the cerebrum as a result of autonomic concomitants secondary to changes in the intermediolateral ceil column.

Most lesions of the motor cortex, especially those caused by a stroke, involve both the motor cortex itself and deeper structures of the cerebrum, especially the basal ganglia. As we said above, if the basal ganglia is unable to perform its requisite functions of modulation there is a resultant production of myospasms. In fact, the degree of basal ganglial lesion and the degree of spasm are directly related.

It is important to point out that the term "lesion" does not necessarily mean "damage." The signs and symptoms of a lesion are produced by any stimuli (or lack thereof) which causes the inability of the postsynaptic tissues to perform their function. In other words, a drive toward potassium equilibrium potential in a fiber that would have otherwise produced a postsynaptic excitatory response, or a drive toward sodium equilibrium in a fiber that produces a postsynaptic inhibitory response will result in the same drive away from threshold in its postsynaptic fiber. Likewise, a drive toward potassium equilibrium potential in a fiber that would have otherwise produced an inhibitory response will result in a drive toward sodium equilibrium potential in its postsynaptic neurons as a result of a lack of inhibition. The end result in each case is that the area involved is unable to perform its proper function, leading to a compromise in the CIS of its postsynaptic tissues, if this takes place throughout the neuraxis as a whole; it becomes compromised, causing it to be functionally dysfunctional.

The motor centers of the brain stem coordinate involuntary postural and positioning reflexes. When these centers have their requisite input of both excitatory and inhibitory stimuli, they are said to be at their functional threshold, and ready to respond adequately to peripheral stimuli, both internal and external.

Essentially, the function of the thalamohypothalamoreticulospinal tract is to inhibit the ipsilateral anterior muscles above T6, and those ipsilateral posterior muscles below T6. Any deafferentation of this tract will tend to drive its CIS toward potassium equilibrium potential and further from threshold, resulting in a concomitant hyperpolarization of its postsynaptic tissues—wherever they are. This creates an inhibition of its inhibitory effect, resulting in an increased tone of the anterior muscles above T6, and an increased tone in the posterior muscles below T6 on the side ipsilateral to the hyperpolarization. As a result, the patient will be unable to meet the demands of simple manual muscle tests such as that of the finger extensors and abductors, and dorsiflexors of the great toe, ipsilaterally. This is the PDW. It is actually a misnomer. It is not a PDW, but rather a hyperpolarization of the extrapyramidal tract that has lost its ability to perform its requisite inhibitory functions which modulate pyramidal influences. This has several structural ramifications, which we will discuss.

The long term effect of the thalamohypothalamoreticulospinal hyperpolarization is a facilitation of those muscles that have lost their natural extrapyramidal inhibition. This leads to an increase in their muscle spindle function and, through monosynaptic facilitation of its alpha and gamma motoneurons, a consequential facilitation of that muscle. Further, through disynaptic postsynaptic inhibitory pathways, the antagonistic muscle becomes defacilitated. This drives the original muscle further toward facilitation, setting up joint pathology with an increased injury potential. Additionally, these same nociceptive pathways are stimulated by polyanionic glycosaminoglycans that arise from the breakdown of joint cartilage. This nociception, together with other aberrant reflexes quicken the production of autonomic concomitants through the interneurons to the intermediolateral ceil column. Further, through crossed extensor reflexes, the contralateral extremities respond in a comparable but converse manner simulating a postural or gait asymmetry. This leads to further nociception and resultant reflexogenic myospasms with a propagation of the pathology of the involved areas.

It is important to realize that the PDW is not primarily one of thalamic hyperpolarization—although that *is* the origin of the thalamohypothalamoreticulospinal outflow—but rather one of cerebellar hyperpolarization as a result of joint mechanoreceptor deafferentation. The thalamic problems are secondary to the cerebellar dysfunction. The cerebellum receives its greatest afferent input from type Ia fibers including those from all joint mechanoreceptors and muscle spindles, both axial and peripheral.

Examples of the diagnostic tests for a PDW are finger and great toe testing, physiologic blind spot evaluation, Romberg's test, finger-to-nose testing, and the evaluation of the ability to perform alternating movements in rapid, smooth and rhythmic succession such as quickly flipping the hands back and forth, and piano type movements.

Finger/Great Toe Testing

One of the best clinical ways to investigate a patient for a PDW is by evaluating the extensors and abductors of their fingers, as well as the dorsiflexors of their great toes. If these muscles are unable to meet the demands of manual muscle testing, it can be said that this patient has a high probability of displaying a PDW, which is named for the side of this functional dysfunction.

The finger extensors and abductors as well as the dorsiflexors of the great toe will be functionally inhibited on the ipsilateral side to the PDW as a result of a lack of modulation from the extrapyramidal system upon the pyramidal system.

Have the patient stand facing you. Ask them to hold their hands out in front of them, with their palms down, and their fingers spread as far apart as possible. Gently but firmly use manual muscle testing procedures to evaluate the patient's ability to maintain this abduction by squeezing the index and little fingers together.

Next, have the patient adduct their fingers, with their hands and fingers in full extension, pointing upward. With the same discreet testing procedures, against your testing pressure, evaluate their ability to maintain this position.

Finally, have the patient sit with their feet hanging freely. Ask the patient to dorsiflex their great toes, and examine their ability to maintain that muscle strength by testing those muscles against resistance.

Any inability on the patient's part to resist the demands of manual muscle testing gives a strong indication of the existence of the PDW on the side of these weaknesses. As a result of the thalamic hyperpolarization, there is an inhibition of the normal and ipsilateral modulatory effect of the thalamohypothalamoreticulospinal tract, which normally leads to a dampening of the anterior muscles above T6 and the posterior muscles below T6, ipsilaterally. This display is secondary to an inhibition of the normal modulatory pathways, thereby allowing the facilitation of those muscles that would otherwise have been inhibited, resulting in a PDW, explaining the patient's inability to maintain strength in their finger abductors and extensors, and ipsilateral dorsiflexors of the great toe.

Physiologic Blind Spot Evaluation

The corticobulbar fibers start, out in company with the corticospinal tract and a few of the fibers continue along with the corticospinal system through the pyramids of the medulla. However, as described above, the majority of fibers quickly take a divergent route at the level of the midbrain.

Figure 96: A graphic representation of the physiological blind spot before treatment.

If the extrapyramidal tracts influence the thalamus, and if the thalamus is brought to threshold as a result of all afferents except those of the sense of smell, and if the thalamus is further stimulated as a result of the corticospinal outflow to the thalamus, then the CIS of thalamic afferentation can be represented by the functional level of all those systems which bring the thalamus to threshold. One such area is that of vision, since the visual afferents of the optic nerve first terminate in the contralateral lateral geniculate body of the thalamus.

Should the CIS of the thalamus and therefore the lateral geniculate body be driven more toward potassium equilibrium potential, then the ability to perceive visual input will be decreased. As a result, there is a very high probability that the physiologic blind spot will be larger (or larger) on the contralateral side.

To evaluate the physiologic blind spot, have the patient stand against a vertical surface such as a door or a wall. Hold a piece of paper (8-1/2" X 11") lengthwise against that surface and have the patient put their nose on the other end of the paper.

Next, while the patient maintains that distance (11") from the surface, place the paper flat against that surface and place a small dot in the center of the paper. Have the patient cover their left eye with their left hand. Next ask them to focus their gaze on the small dot throughout the test. Their eye should not wander from that spot. With a sharp pencil, slowly move the pencil toward the right and ask the patient to tell you when the tip of the pencil disappears. When it does, place a dot, and continue laterally until the patient recognizes the tip of the pencil returns. Place another dot. Next, return to the center of that: area of physiological blindness and move the pencil upward until the patient again notices the tip of the pencil. Place another dot. Finally, go back to the center of the area and do the same thing, moving your pencil toward the bottom of the paper. Place a dot when the patient notices the tip of the pencil. The four dots can now be connected and represents the physiologic blind spot for that eye.

Now do the same thing for the left eye. Have the patient maintain the same distance from the paper. Have them cover the right eye with their right hand, and proceed as above, but in the opposite direction.

Figure 97: A graphic representation of the physiological blind spot after treatment.

A person with a hyperpolarized thalamus will show a difference in size from one physiologic blind spot to the other. The side of the larger physiologic blind spot represents the side opposite to that of the hyperpolarized thalamus (since the optic nerve decussates at the optic chiasma). And, it gives a pictorial representation of the degree of input from all areas that have synaptic contact with that thalamus.

Autonomic Concomitants

Those postsynaptic projections of the thalamohypothalamoreticulospinal tract ultimately make contact with the intermediolateral cell column. Since the intermediolateral cell column is responsible for the disynaptic postsynaptic inhibition of nociceptive reflexogenic efferents in the anterior horn via its interneurons, the hyperpolarization of this area also explains the production of the autonomic concomitants.

A PDW can be accompanied by several autonomic concomitants. The corticothalamohypothalamoreticulospinal pathway constitutes an extrapyramidal pathway by which motor regions of the cortex can act on the spinal motor apparatus. The physiological role of the projections from sensory regions of the cerebral cortex to reticulospinal neurons is less certain, but such pathways may be involved in the regulation of sensory input to the spinal cord through reticular-evoked presynaptic inhibition of spinal afferent fibers, or through postsynaptic inhibition of spinal sensory interneurons. At the same time, this same pathway conveys autonomic modulation from the Edinger-Westphal nucleus of the third cranial nerve at its most rostral extent through the intermediolateral cell column, which terminates in the sacral portions of the cord at S2-4 to influence among other things, dilation of the pupils, respiration, circulation, sweating, shivering, etc.

Posture and Gait

Skeletal motor neurons are commonly referred to as the "final common pathway," because they integrate all CNS activity controlling a given muscle—from spindle afferent fibers, spinal interneurons involved in spinal reflexes, brainstem nuclei and cortical pyramidal cells. The function of the reflexes is to influence the neuronal signal (Table 27), or in other words, modulate the interplay of one area with another. This can only happen, if you recall, if the reflex is brought to threshold. If it has been driven more toward potassium equilibrium potential (or away from threshold), then the modulatory control cannot occur resulting in nociceptive reflexogenic efferents as a consequence of deafferentation.

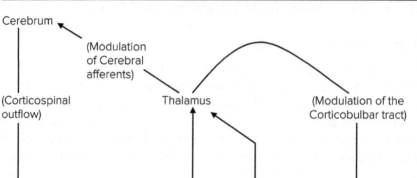

Table 27: SCHEMATIC OF NEURONAL FLOW

When a person transitions their step from one foot to the other, it requires a series of stereotyped postural adjustments to be set in motion. This involves a shift of body weight from one side to the other and from back to front where the weight is born principally by the nonreaching foot and managed through the motion of the contralateral hand.

Try to imagine the impact on functional status if reflexes are not brought to threshold. This, in itself, represents a deafferentation of some presynaptic area that has been driven toward potassium equilibrium potential, resulting in the hyperpolarization of a function that should be modulating its postsynaptic stimuli. As a result, that function is freely allowed to do that which it should be modulated to perform.

Exercises

A patient who demonstrates a PDW needs to be treated not only with specialized fast-stretch coupled chiropractic manual manipulative techniques, but also certain specific exercises (Tables 28 and 29) in order to facilitate the specific cerebellar hyperpolarization and its resultant thalamic drive toward potassium equilibrium potential, and to avoid further facilitation of the contralateral side of the cerebellum, which has already been driven toward sodium equilibrium, and thereby depolarized.

In order to cause unilateral facilitation of the hyperpolarized thalamus contralateral to the cerebellar deafferentation secondary to a deafferentation of the joint mechanoreceptors, the patient must do only those exercises which encourages facilitation of: 1) The anterior muscles of the upper extremity on the side contralateral to the PDW, 2) The posterior muscles of the upper extremity on the side ipsilateral to the PDW, 3) The facilitation of those anterior muscles of the lower extremity on the side ipsilateral to the PDW, and, 4) The facilitation of those posterior muscles of the lower extremity on the side contralateral to the PDW.

For example: A patient with a hyperpolarization of the right cerebellum will present with a left PDW as a result of the thalamic hyperpolarization. They display a right foot forward gait pattern with the left arm forward and the head turned toward the right.

The patient's structural compromise is a result of the left thalamic hyperpolarization secondary to a decreased CIS of the right cerebellum and a zygapophyseal joint mechanoreceptor deafferentation, with a consequential and concomitant increase in the size of the right physiologic blind spot.

In the left PDW, the muscles of a neurologically neutral posture will be functionally facilitated and functionally inhibited consistent with the right foot forward gait pattern even though the patient may appear to be physically standing in the anatomically neutral position. As a result, each of the joints connected by these muscles will be drawn toward the facilitation and limited through the opposite direction, creating further deafferentation. It is important to keep in mind that we are discussing a neurologic posture, not necessarily a structurally visible variant from a plumb line (although that may be present also).

The left PDW is best treated by exercising the right anterior and left posterior neck muscles, the extensors of the left upper extremity, flexors of the right upper extremity, anterior thigh and dorsiflexors of the great toe on the left lower extremity, and the posterior thigh and plantar flexors of the right lower extremity.

Further, the patient should do no flexion exercises with the left side of their neck, or extension exercises with the right side of their neck; no flexion exercises of the left upper extremity; no extension exercises of the right upper extremity; no extension exercises of the left posterior thigh muscles or plantar flexors of its great toe; no flexion exercises of the anterior thigh muscles of the right lower extremity or dorsiflexors of its great toe. To do these exercises would facilitate the left cerebellum and consequently the right thalamus and encourage the PDW, causing further exaggeration of the patient's physiologic blind spot and dysfunctional gait mechanisms. In other words, doing these exercises could exercise the patient right into their PDW and its concomitants.

The "Struggle Bug" Exercise

The patient can do some simple exercises at home that are essentially a modified cross-crawl exercise, but with specificity determined by the side of pyramidal weakness; it is called "the Struggle Bug" exercise. Consistent with the left PDW, have the patient lie on their back with their right thigh flexed at the hip and left arm flexed with their hand closed on their chest. This represents the right foot forward gait. Tell the patient that you want them to do *five things at once*: 1) extend their left arm with their palm up, 2) flex the right arm with their hand closed on their chest, 3) extend the right leg, 4) flex the left leg, and 5) turn their head to the left. (The opposite procedure works for a right PDW.) These movements must be done slowly with purposeful movement.

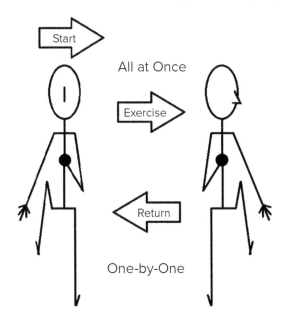

Figure 98: Left Pyramidal Distribution of Weakness.
This exercise is to be done very s-l-o-w-l-y for a
minimum of 5 minutes twice daily.

Once the movement is complete, the patient should return to the original posture by moving each of the five areas *one by one*, but there is no specific order. The return to the start posture is as important as the exercise itself. If the patient were to return to their start posture with one movement they would be mimicking the gait pattern they are working to extinguish, essentially potentiating the contralateral thalamus and cerebellum and allowing the hyperpolarization to persist.

Explain to the patient that the muscles consistent with each gait pattern are functionally facilitated and inhibited consistent with that posture. Whereas, the patient may be able to stand in the anatomical position, the pyramidal pattern is one of "stroke antalgia."

Figure 98 is an example of an exercise that is used to rehabilitate a left PDW. Here is what I tell the patient as I describe the exercise:

> *"You start with your left arm flexed and your right knee flexed. Your right arm is straight and your hand is palm down and open and your left leg are flat. This is your start position.*

The exercise is done all at once, but let me tell you what I want you to do before you do it. I want you to bend your left knee and straighten out your right knee at the same time; they just trade places. At the same time I want you to bend your right elbow and close your hand on your chest. At the same time you are going to straighten out your left elbow and open your hand palm down on the table (or the surface they are laying on, a bed, the floor or somewhere else). Finally, and at the same time I want you to turn your head to the left. In this exercise your head never turns to the right.

Now, think about what you are going to do: switch your legs and your arms and turn your head to the left all at the same time. Whenever you are ready go ahead and do it S-L-O-W-L-Y."

Now the patient does the exercise and you tell them to stop. Continue your explanation with: *"To come back to the start position again you do exactly the opposite movements but only one at a time, and there is no special sequence."* Then I count out loud as they patient does the movement to reinforce that there are five individual movements that must be done one at a time.

Have them try the exercise again slowly until they feel more comfortable with the movements. Then explain to them, *"If I had five people standing here in the room and I wanted them to all clap at the same time so I only heard one clap, do you think they could do it together on their first try?"* You will hear different replies, but the point is that it would probably take practice. *"Pretend that the left knee is one clap (and I physically touch that knee as I am explaining this procedure) and the right knee is a second clap, the right arm is clap number three, the left arm is clap number four, and the head is clap number five. Now you try it and I want you to do it so I only hear one clap!"* And let the patient try the exercise again, but reinforce that it is to be done slowly. Give them several tries again so that they are more comfortable with the movement.

Finally, describe to the patient, *"In the normal walking gait the first movement is with the head. The head actually moves before the arms and legs move. So you should initiate your exercise with your head and let your arms and legs follow."* While you are standing there, show the patient what it looks like to initiate the movement with your head and let your arms follow with extension of the arm on the side toward head rotation and flexion of the arm on the side opposite head rotation. (Recall that this is the same movement as seen with the tonic neck reflex; walking demonstrates the tonic neck reflex.) Then watch them do it. Let them do several series of exercises while you watch and be sure to count with them and for them as they return to the start position one by one.

As far as individual muscle exercise is concerned, Tables 27 and 28 suggest specific exercises to rehabilitate the left and right PDW. These exercises should only be done after the patient's specific aerobic base is firmly established relative to their metabolic and target heart rates. Further, these tables are only suggestions because any other related muscle can also be exercised, and be sure that other muscles are exercised according to their related pyramidal posture. After the exercise, be sure to give the exercised muscle a short (up to 20 seconds) stretch as that will help to build greater myofibril interconnectivity in the muscle and follow that with a long (40 seconds) stretch to its antagonist.

Figure 99 represents another example of a pyramidal exercise, but this time it is relative to a right PDW. The movements and exercise are essentially the same but obviously the explanation switches right for left.

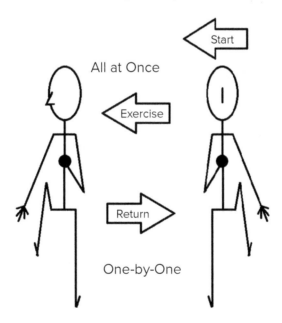

Figure 99: Left Pyramidal Distribution of Weakness. This exercise is to be done very s-l-o-w-l-y for a minimum of 5 minutes twice daily.

Treatment

The best way to treat neuromusculoskeletal issues related to the PDW is to direct a fast stretch coupled chiropractic manual manipulative adjustive thrust toward those joints demonstrating a resistance to movement on the side contralateral to the hyperpolarization of the thalamohypothalamoreticulospinal tract, or ipsilateral to the side of cerebellar deafferentation. A slow stretch or uncoupled thrust directed toward those same joints will only serve to further stabilize the already fixated joints through the stimulation of the Ia afferents from muscle spindles, and lead to an increased degenerative potential with the consequential production of polyanionic glycosaminoglycans and nociception. Faulty rib mechanics further contribute to the cerebellar and thalamic hyperpolarization through these same tracts. This leads to the thalamohypothalamoreticulospinal dysfunction, and a clinical state of hypoxia, which may result in changes in cellular stability with resultant free radical production, as well as changes in systemic pH, and other homeostatic instabilities.

Consequently, the patient might also benefit from supplemental oxygen therapy to provide the substrate necessary to rebuild mitochondrial electron acceptors to facilitate cellular membrane replacement. Further, certain specific nutrients should be provided to enhance the metabolic processes, produce ATP, allow for more purposeful protein replication and provide for the ability to scavenge for free radicals.

It is advisable for the patient to utilize upper body motion with a device like an Cybex Upper Body Ergorneter (UBE) in order to provide the isokinetic activity necessary to facilitate the spinocerebellar and cuneocerebellar afferents to the cerebellar centers, thereby stimulating the proper supraspinal modulatory events necessary to increase bony co-adaptation and stabilize the series elastic elements of the paraspinal system.

After stabilization of the aerobic base and once the PDW has been resolved, the patient will also benefit from an aerobic exercise program directed toward rebuilding the series elastic elements of the paraspinal system. This is necessary in order to rehabilitate the muscle necessary for the development of endurance activity, and to provide for a greater quantum of bony co-adaptation and the resultant zygapophyseal afferentation.

If the PDW does not resolve in a reasonable period of time, this patient would probably benefit from the application of a full body cast, shoulder to hips, including one thigh. This is necessary in order to isolate the side of the PDW and cause a state of selective atrophy in those muscles that have become functionally facilitated. In the case of a left PDW, the cast should be applied with the isolation of the left lower extremity at the thigh. It is advisable for the patient to use the UBE at the same time as the full body cast.

Summary

The simple elimination of one or two of the symptoms of a PDW is not enough to say the treatment was a success. Because the human nervous system is multimodal, the elimination of one set of symptoms may cause the exacerbation of another set of symptoms that are either related or unrelated to the first set of symptoms.

The PDW is a very common finding in the great majority of chiropractic patients. It can be responsible for many of the most common symptoms ranging from mild autonomic dysfunctions to the most bizarre cases of structural compromise that respond slowly at best. Routinely, this kind of patient is the one who is told they "have a disc" pathology, and is referred out for surgery. When the procedures discussed in this paper are applied in an appropriate mariner, these cases respond predictably without surgical intervention.

The mark of successful treatment is a functional resolution of each of the examination findings mentioned above, and an increase in the CIS of the neuraxis as a whole. Reexamination should show a strengthening of the finger extensors and abductors and the dorsiflexors of the great toe, a balancing of the physiologic blind spots, a normalization of the neurological posture, a steadying of the cerebellar functions as well as the elimination of the autonomic concomitants and pain.

Suggested Exercises

Left Pyramidal Distribution of Weakness (Right Foot Forward Gait)

Table 28: EXERCISES FOR LEFT PYRAMIDAL DISTRIBUTION OF WEAKNESS			
Extremity	**Weight Training**	**Short Stretches**	**Long Stretch**
RIGHT UPPER (Above T6)	SCM	SCM	
	Pectoralis major	Pectoralis major	Shoulder extensors
	Ant. Deltoid	Ant. Deltoid	Latissimus dorsi
	Biceps	**Biceps**	**Triceps**
	Internal rotators	Internal rotators	External rotators
	Wrist flexors	Wrist flexors	Wrist extensors
	Finger adductors	Finger adductors	
LEFT UPPER (Above T6)	Upper trapezius	Upper trapezius	
	Triceps	**Triceps**	**Biceps**
	Rhomboids	Rhomboids	Pectoralis major
	Latissimus dorsi	Latissimus dorsi	Deltoid
	Teres Minor	Teres minor	Internal rotators
	Wrist extensors	Wrist extensors	Wrist flexors
	Finger abductors	Finger abductors	
RIGHT LOWER (Below T6)	**Hamstrings**	**Hamstrings**	**Quadriceps**
	Piriformis	Piriformis	Internal rotators
	Abductors	Abductors	Adductors
	TFL	TFL	Adductors
	Foot plantar flexors	Foot plantar flexors	Foot dorsiflexors
LEFT LOWER (Below T6)	Adductors	Adductors	Abductors
	Quadriceps	**Quadriceps**	**Hamstrings**
	Abdominals	Abdominals	
	Foot dorsiflexors	Foot dorsiflexors	Foot plantar flexors

(NOTE: The bold print signifies those muscles with which most people are generally familiar. Other muscles can and should be added to this list to individualize the results.)

Suggested Exercises

Right Pyramidal Distribution of Weakness (Left Foot Forward Gait)

Table 29: EXERCISES FOR RIGHT PYRAMIDAL DISTRIBUTION OF WEAKNESS			
Extremity	Weight Training	Short Stretches	Long Stretch
LEFT UPPER (Above T6)	SCM	SCM	
	Pectoralis major	Pectoralis major	Shoulder extensors
	Ant. Deltoid	Ant. Deltoid	Latissimus dorsi
	Biceps	**Biceps**	**Triceps**
	Internal rotators	Internal rotators	External rotators
	Wrist flexors	Wrist flexors	Wrist extensors
	Finger adductors	Finger adductors	
RIGHT UPPER (Above T6)	Upper trapezius	Upper trapezius	
	Triceps	**Triceps**	**Biceps**
	Rhomboids	Rhomboids	Pectoralis major
	Latissimus dorsi	Latissimus dorsi	Deltoid
	Teres Minor	Teres minor	Internal rotators
	Wrist extensors	Wrist extensors	Wrist flexors
	Finger abductors	Finger abductors	
LEFT LOWER (Below T6)	**Hamstrings**	**Hamstrings**	**Quadriceps**
	Piriformis	Piriformis	Internal rotators
	Abductors	Abductors	Adductors
	TFL	TFL	Adductors
	Foot plantar flexors	Foot plantar flexors	Foot dorsiflexors
RIGHT LOWER (Below T6)	Adductors	Adductors	Abductors
	Quadriceps	**Quadriceps**	**Hamstrings**
	Abdominals	Abdominals	
	Foot dorsiflexors	Foot dorsiflexors	Foot plantar flexors

(NOTE: The bold print signifies those muscles with which most people are generally familiar. Other muscles can and should be added to this list to individualize the results.)

277

Definitions relative to a pyramidal display:

1. Pyramidal distribution of weakness: increased facilitation of the anterior muscles above T6, and an increased facilitation of the posterior muscles below T6; there may be symptoms of autonomic concomitants.

2. Hyperpolarized: A tissue whose functional state is depressed from threshold.

3. Central integrative state (CIS): The state of function of a tissue that is derived as a result of the sum of all excitatory and inhibitory input to that tissue,

4. Neuraxis: The nervous system from the peripheral nerves to the cerebrum.

5. Deafferentation: A decrease in the number of afferent signals being sent to a specific area as a result of a limited range of motion.

6. Potassium equilibrium potential: An increase in intracellular potassium with a consequential drive away from threshold; a state of depressed function.

7. Spatial summation: The sum of all the afferent input from the surrounding neuronal activity.

8. Temporal summation: The sum of all the afferent input from the surrounding neuronal activity within a given period of time.

9. Depolarization: A tissue whose functional state is driven more toward threshold and is in an increased state of readiness to respond.

10. Nociceptive reflexogenic efferents: The motor response to pain that results in myospasm and increased joint destabilization.

11. Polyanionic glycosaminoglycans: Specific biochemicals that arise as a result of the breakdown of joint cartilage.

12. Sodium equilibrium potential: An increase in intracellular sodium with a consequential drive toward threshold; a state of increased function.

13. Series elastic elements: The muscle(s), bones, nerves and blood vessels that compose a joint.

Summary of Receptor Based Solutions™

Managing the Functional Display to
a Constantly Changing Environment

The human nervous system is sensory dependent with an inborn preprogrammed response to our constantly changing one-G environment. It is that simple. But in its simplicity the human nervous system is purely intricate. Understanding the natural refinements of human magnificence, as my mentor and personal friend Dr. Ted Carrick describes it, is not always so easy.

The fundamental matrix of the human design can be found in the primitive reflexes. Their clinical display is well documented, but their clinical significance has, until now, been limited to infants and toddlers, and older pathological adults. Between these two extremes there appeared to be no reason for involving primitive reflexes in the standard neurological examination. However, we now know that there is, in fact, a clinical reality for the use of these functional reflexes in daily practice.

Receptors are the Foundation

The perception of human function starts with the receptors and never ends. Understanding the majesty of what it means to be fully human is a lifelong quest. It cannot be learned in a weekend seminar or from a single book; not even a collection of papers written by one who has been at the quest all their life. There is always something new and always a new way to perceive the human condition.

It can be said that health is the freedom to live and move in a fully human manner without hindrance. But relative to that definition, who among us is truly healthy? Nobody. Our existence in this one-G environment makes us prone to structural problems that show up in our structure, both frame and muscle. Deafferentation is at the source of most health conditions, and it is not related to pain; pain often comes later. Finding the source of deafferentation and then correcting it is the key to helping a person regain and then maintain their health.

Each functional reflex arrangement begins with the receptors and has its impact upon the efferent response if it is challenged using MMT as functional neurology—fMMT. Having a patient sit on the examining table and testing the usual deep tendon reflex by sharply tapping the patellar tendon with a reflex hammer and observing the response has clinical value. However, tapping that same tendon of the supine patient and then checking the functional response of the isolated rectus femoris muscle adds an enormous level of clinically valuable. It may show one response seated and a different response supine.

Another valuable fMMT is testing the muscles of a patient in any posture and then having them turn their head in one direction or the other to demonstrate the functional response to cervical mechanoreceptor stimulation; i.e., the ATNR test. The supine response is well known in the infant, but any response other than that which is considered to be normal should be considered pathological no matter what the person's posture or age. These normal and abnormal displays are clinically important to know and apply in daily clinical practice.

The tonic labyrinthine, flexor withdrawal, Galant (with all its newly discovered and highly applicable variants, such as the Modified and Upper Galant Reflexes), crossed extensor, tonic lumbar reflexes and their associated cortical release involvement are all clinically essential if the doctor truly desires to understand the functional state of his or her patient and what to do to ease their condition.

The point is that any one of these functional reflexes can be evaluated in any postural state—upright, sitting, or dependent— with the understanding that each indicates a different neurological response to gravity and the resolution of these findings may need a specific gravitational influence for correction.

Human movement is a beautiful gift. Its majesty should be one of the primary quests of any doctor who truly desires the long term health and wellness of their patients. Applying these tests on a regular basis and describing their involvement to your patients will open up a new world of understanding to doctor and patient alike.

Make Time for Health

I once saw a shirt that had writing on the back complaining about the aspirin this person took for their headache that was caused by the medication they took for hay fever that developed as a result of another drug they took for an uneasy stomach caused by the Ritalin they took for a short attention span, etc. This shirt went on and on with other conditions that resulted from a different drug they took for something else. The gist was that all these medications were because exercise, a good diet and regular chiropractic care are just too much trouble.

The right kind of chiropractic adjustments—coupled manual manipulation of those spine and spinal related structures that have a limited motion—stimulate neurological function in a way that no other therapy can match. If a person takes drugs because of their limited attention span, well, functional neurology has a better answer. Rather than bathing the brain and other vital areas with the side effects of the medications used to block the symptoms of the problem, the right neurological application will directly affect the source of neurological deafferentation and bring about the functional state that is most appropriate for that person. There are not side effects to a functional neurological treatment delivered in the right way.

The centerline spine and its associated neurological structures form the foundation of both organization and function of optimal human performance. A sound functional base starts in the structural centerline—the spine and CNS. The two are functionally linked and whatever happens to the one directly affects the other. If the centerline structure breaks down then so does the centerline brain, and vice versa.

Bipedal posture and gait are among the unique traits of human ability. It all depends upon the receptor input from each side of the body, and the centerline nervous system—the cerebellum, basal ganglia, thalamus, among other centerline structures—is the key to comparing and contrasting that input. When the centerline centers are properly afferentated then the more rostral and caudal structures are nourished with the neurological stimulation that feeds them. However, when deafferentation creeps in these core centers have to involve more resources to compare the errors and both structural and functional dysfunction is the eventual outcome. When the neurological hierarchy is compromised, then the symptoms of sickness and disease that would have otherwise been kept under control are the result.

The breakdown of the centerline structures work their way into peripheral tissues, and these peripheral structures can also work their way centrally. There is no way around the postural breakdown that accompanies dysfunctional conditions. Structure and function are directly linked. Once a tissue's function is compromised it must be rehabilitated in order to avoid further degenerative change, and the rehabilitation has to be done consistent with the functional breakdown in order to not exceed the capacity of the system as a whole.

Think of it this way, if one has a balanced system, a balanced diet will help maintain their health. But if that person has a vitamin deficiency taking a multiple vitamin will only maintain that deficiency. It makes more sense to meet that nutrient need by supplying that needed vitamin and then maintain the balance with a balanced nutrient. It is no different with rehabilitation. If a person has a postural imbalance, working both sides equally will only serve to make the stronger muscle stronger at the expense of the weaker muscle that tries to keep up with the stronger muscle but eventually fails, giving up its counterbalance that only leads to further imbalance.

Serving mankind in the finest way involves understanding the wonder of the human nervous system. Giving a drug or having surgery are seldom the way to treat the human condition. Granted, sometimes drugs and/or surgery are necessary in order to save a person's life, but most of the time a functional neurological remedy is the most appropriate way to serve our fellow human beings best.

Make time for health.

Stay well!

Case Study #13

History and Presenting Complaints: Eileen, 16; loves to play water polo. She complained of pain on the inside of her left knee with every kick as she circumducts her left leg medially while treading water.

Exam Findings: During the course of a normal physical examination it was observed that the following muscles appeared to be unable to meet the demands of manual muscle testing, bilaterally: rectus femoris, psoas major, sartorius, gluteus medius, tensor fascia lata, hamstrings, piriformis, and popliteus, all of which involve her knees.

The rectus femoris appeared to be functionally inhibited bilaterally without functional facilitation upon tapping the distal aspect of the rectus femoris ipsilaterally. Further, the rectus femoris appeared to be functionally inhibited bilaterally with functional facilitation upon tapping the origin of the rectus femoris, ipsilaterally.

The psoas major appeared to be functionally inhibited without facilitation with the patient's head rotated contralaterally, but with facilitation with the patient's head rotated ipsilaterally. The sartorius appeared to be functionally inhibited bilaterally without functional facilitation with the patient's head rotated contralaterally. The gluteus medius appeared to be functionally inhibited bilaterally without functional facilitation with the patient's head rotated ipsilaterally, but with facilitation with the patient's head rotated contralaterally. The tensor fascia lata appeared to be functionally inhibited without functional facilitation with the patient's head rotated ipsilaterally, but with facilitation with the patient's head rotated contralaterally. The popliteus appeared to be functionally inhibited without facilitation with the patient's head rotated ipsilaterally.

Stroking the sole of the patient's foot with a sharp object appeared to cause inhibition of the rectus femoris ipsilaterally with a concomitant facilitation of the hamstrings contralaterally.

In the prone posture, the hamstrings appeared to be functionally inhibited bilaterally without functional facilitation upon tapping the deep tendon reflex at its origin and/or insertion ipsilaterally, but with facilitation when stroking the Galant reflex contralaterally. The piriformis appeared to be functionally inhibited bilaterally without functional facilitation with the patient's head rotated ipsilaterally, but with facilitation when stroking the Galant reflex ipsilaterally.

Clinical Impression: The patient's functional condition appears to be contrary to structural stability with a demonstrable dysfunction of her reflexive performance.

Treatment Plan: The patient will receive coupled chiropractic manual manipulative procedures to her spine and spinal related structures in order to cure or relieve her condition and reestablish normal neurophysiological responses. She will also receive structural rehabilitation exercises consistent with her treatments.

Response to Care: Immediately after treatment the patient experienced a relief of her knee pain.

Discussion: The patient's pain was the result of her inability to presynaptically inhibit nociceptive reflexogenic afferents in the dorsal aspect of her spinal cord. As a result, she had pain with every knee movement. Reestablishing the normal reciprocal movements necessary for increased joint stability returned the normal and preprogrammed human movement parameters with a concomitant reduction of pain.

Frequently Asked Questions

1. Q: What is Functional Neurology?

    A: A good friend of mine just told me that his patient said, "You rebooted my brain!"

    This whole idea of functional neurology began within the chiropractic community as an alternative holistic specialty that deals with the functional instability of the brain and the entire nervous system, but is quickly attracting those with more traditional medical training.

    The original concepts of functional neurology were developed by my good friend and teacher, Professor Frederick Carrick, of the Carrick Institute for Graduate Studies in Cape Canaveral, Florida. Prof. Carrick's wisdoms have progressed relative to his vast clinical experience, innovative research, and continuing deeper understanding of the human nervous system's function.

    Functional neurologists receive specialized training in the neurological sciences. These specialists are skilled at stimulating a person's sensory input and monitoring the changes in their neurological response. They treat each patient according to what would be normal; if the patient's systems were working right, they would respond in an anticipated manner. If these systems respond abnormally, then the treatment changes and the new response is observed. These diagnostic procedures are designed to detect and treat functional neurological changes before their adaptive progression to irreversible pathology. The goal is to restore optimal function for health and wellness, to improve autonomic balance, return hormone stability, encourage immune display, and reduce the experience of pain.

The art and science of functional neurology is the multidisciplinary study of the dynamics of a person's neurological function within the context of their greater health. It considers that a person's functional state is generally determined by the quality of their brain's input and the clarity of its output as well as the supply of oxygen and the essential components for repair that reach that person's nervous system.

Functional neurologists consider that the functional state of a person's nervous system will impact all embryologically and anatomically related systems. Since all these systems are related, they use these relationships to effect a positive neurological change that builds functional neuroplasticity within the dysfunctioning nervous system, thus improving the neuronal performance of the whole person.

2. Q: You have many letters behind your name; this represents an enormous amount of time and study. How does this serve you?

   A: Just as with any professional who has letter designations after their name, each set represents a level of education in an area of specialty. This education teaches me how to do things right. Better yet, it serves my patients because I have spent the time necessary to study and understand the art and science of natural healthcare and the specialties I have chosen. I am always working to improve the level of service I provide, and that includes regular educational updates at various places around the world from the healthcare professionals who can teach at that level. And believe me I have had some of the world's best teachers!

3. Q: As a functional neurologist, what skill set or understandings would you like to see other professionals and ancillary support practitioners, i.e., Rolfers and the Structural Integration Community for example, have to support your work?

   A: I believe a working understanding of neurology is important. I think it is important for other doctors as well as those therapists who do body work to realize how to apply their understanding at increasingly higher levels. I would encourage them to always strive to better understand the basics but do not settle for that level of understanding. Strive for more. Challenge yourself.

4. Q: (A similar question) What place does massage therapy, structural integration have in affecting, altering or supporting functional neurology?

    A: Whenever one person places their hands on another person with the intent to treat some misalignment it is important that they do it right. Understanding how the muscles—in the case of a massage therapist or structural integration therapist—send signals to the brain and how the brain uses these signals to make the muscles respond can make the difference between functional stability and functional breakdown. Many people go see a massage therapist for relaxation when in fact that may be the exact opposite of what may be needed. I am not saying that a person should sometimes be massaged to tighten their muscles, but if the brain is causing an increased muscle tone in order to hold some adaptation necessary for brain stability, the last thing you would want to do is to relax that tone. That can make the difference between a healthy brain and one that breaks down too quickly.

5. Q: With a better understanding of functional neurology, what unique opportunities do you see that we, as Rolfers, may have to influence the neurological health of our clients?

    A: This question expands on the previous one. A greater understanding of functional neurology will help you perceive your client's condition much faster. I am talking about more than their muscles and body posture. If a therapist can functionally realize that a person's posture is an expression of their brain's functional level and how that brain function is affecting the person as a whole, that therapist can go much further in their application than just realizing that there is postural imbalance. It's not all about relaxing muscles to make joints move more.

6. Q: How do you define posture? Postural displays? How do you as a functional neurologist determine these displays with your patients? How do these displays relate to brain imbalance?

    A: This is a very important question and one of the main reasons for writing this book. Posture is a function of brain and the consequence of that person's nervous system relative to gravity. There are many pathways that give input to the brain relative to its internal and external environment. Are these pathways intact?

Are they sending an adequate signal to provoke an appropriate response? Are the component parts of the brain and the brain as a whole healthy enough to respond appropriately to the input it receives? The answers to all these questions and many others ultimately display themselves in the contraction of a muscle. To the level that the doctor or therapist understands and treats these issues properly the patient will receive benefit.

7. Q: From the functional neurology viewpoint, what initiates the fibrotic cascade that forms adhesions we find in our clients?

A: One of the keys to better understand the whole concept of adhesions is found in the greater application of the immune response related to inflammatory changes. The fibrotic cascade begins with an initial epithelial insult and gradually progresses to a complex series of biological processes that involve systems as deep as the cellular level.

Functional neurology provides a greater understanding of the roles that inflammatory cells play in the fibrotic process and where to apply new points of therapeutic intervention. The application of this knowledge helps us to induce a shift from a pro-fibrotic microenvironment to an anti-fibrotic microenvironment.

8. Q: Would you comment on adaptive shortening as a result of exceeding metabolic capacity

A: Adaptive shortening is the idea that a muscle can adapt its functional resting length to the length that that muscle is habitually used or positioned. Adaptive shortening is a muscle response to a spinal cord consequence as a result of reciprocal breakdown. As the metabolic capacity of a system adapts to its level of function the consequence is a reduced ability to function at higher levels and the system consequentially fatigues at a faster pace.

9. Q: I know you work with Rolfers and other allied professionals. How do you utilize Rolfers in your practice?

A: Anybody who works on a patient or client must be aware that their work has central consequences. That is, any stimulus from the outside will provoke neurological changes that have their consequence in the brain. It may seem benign to work a muscle and see it change its function, but one must always remember that any change in muscle function is always the result of a change in brain function, first. The human brain is very plastic; it will respond to the stimulation it receives because it is receptor dependent. What is muscle work besides receptor stimulation? Stimulating primary afferents modifies the motor response. That changed motor response is modified for better or for worse, but when it changes for the worse it is consistent with derogatory brain changes—including nerve cell death—and that can never be good for the patient.

10. Q: What skills do Rolfers have that support your practice?

A: The only Rolfers that assist my patients are those who I can tell have a fundamental grasp of the neurological consequences of central integration. I will not allow just anyone to work with my patients. I have my assistants read tens of books and I literally spent hundreds of hours in detailed discussion with anyone that works in my office on my patients. I even caution my patients against outside massage unless I talk with the massage therapist first.

11. Q: Please explain facilitation and inhibition (modulation).

A: This is a good fundamental question. A muscle's normal activity is a combination of contraction and relaxation, technically referred to as facilitation and inhibition, respectively. When the nervous system is stimulated to cause facilitation or inhibition upon demand of some outside provocation we say that the muscle response has changed functionally or conditionally; these terms are interchangeable. So we can say that a muscle has functional facilitation or functional inhibition; conditional facilitation or conditional inhibition.

The functional facilitation and/or functional inhibition of a muscle—its modulation—has to do with the quality of communication between the brain and that muscle. It refers to the capacity of a muscle to contract or relax fully upon demand and in a timely manner.

Muscle facilitation and inhibition are caused by a number of variables. In fact, there are several scenarios that lead to functional muscle responses. When we use the words functional facilitation and/or functional inhibition, they relate to the muscle's modified ability to send and receive neural information. It does not mean that the muscle is unable to relax or contract, only that its ability to contract or relax on demand is modified.

12. Q: Can you differentiate muscle strength from facilitation?

A: The human body is wrought with asymmetry and therefore normal variations exist in muscle function and strength even in the same person. Take for example the muscle differences in a person who favors one side of their body relative to the other; we see this all the time. This scenario is relative asymmetry. Those muscles on this person's dominant side often are stronger than the same muscles on the other side of their body, but both are facilitated if they are working; both have tone.

If we build on the discussion above, differentiating muscle strength from facilitation cannot be easily evaluated using X-rays, CAT scans or MRIs, or other high-tech devices. However, it is possible to measure the strength and facilitation with manual muscle testing. In general, a "strong" muscle can be measured relative to a "weaker" one.

People often define muscle balance and imbalance in terms of strength, making it more a local phenomenon that reflects muscular exercise. The problem is that too much or too little strength in one muscle or muscle group compared to another can cause facilitation of that stronger muscle, which imbalances the muscles on the other side of a joint leading to further imbalance.

A sailboat's mast stands square because the cables on either side of the mast pull with equal strength. The same is true of a bone between two muscles; a joint is stable because the muscles have a balanced pull on the structure. If muscles develop an imbalance then the joint gets pulled toward the tighter muscle. An example of this can be seen with weight lifting if the hamstrings are exercised more than quadriceps. The result is that the hamstrings become much stronger relative to the quadriceps. This could make the knee and/or hip joint more vulnerable to injury.

The cause of exercise imbalance can occur from improper weight training, one-sided sports—such as golf and racquet sports, etc.—or having a job that requires a high level of physical activity in only one muscle or muscle group compared to the same muscle or group of muscles on the other side of the body. These are examples of using one muscle—or group of muscles—while reducing the action of another muscle or group of muscles causing imbalance. The lack of strength, typically from a sedentary lifestyle, can also contribute to muscle imbalance. These are examples of muscles that are strong or facilitated, but there is imbalance and structural weakness.

13. Q: What are the muscle types and their metabolism?

A: There are three types of muscle tissue—cardiac, smooth, and skeletal. Cardiac muscle cells are located in the walls of the heart. They appear striated and are under involuntary control. Smooth muscle fibers are found in walls of all hollow visceral organs except the heart. They appear spindle-shaped, and are also under involuntary control. Skeletal muscle fibers are found in muscles that are attached to the skeleton. They are appearance is striated—marked with parallel grooves, ridges, stripes, or narrow bands—but these muscles are under voluntary control. Skeletal muscles are the body's most abundant tissue, comprising about 23% of a woman's body weight and about 40% of a man's body weight.

There are two general skeletal muscle types relative to their metabolism: there are red and white muscles; aerobic and anaerobic types, respectively. The red muscles are also known as slow twitch (type I) muscles that are endowed with abundant mitochondria. Aerobic muscles are more efficient at using oxygen to generate more fuel (known as ATP) for continuous, extended useful work over long periods before they fatigue. They fire slower than fast twitch fibers.

The white muscles—fast twitch (type II) muscles—are much better at generating short bursts of strength or speed than slow muscles. Fast twitch fibers fire faster and generally produce the same amount of force per contraction as slow twitch muscles, hence their name. On average, human muscles contain a genetic balance of slow and fast twitch fibers in most of the muscles used for movement.

14. Q: How are these red and white muscle types affected by brain imbalance and their related postural display?

A: The aerobic muscles are more related to antigravity muscle function and upright posture. The paraspinal muscles, for example, are plentifully endowed with mitochondria that allow the spine and all of its centerline attachments to generate the richest signal to the brain. However, any breakdown of the involuntary signal to these midline muscles secondary to some cerebellar deafferentation can lead to the subluxation of these structures thereby reducing the muscle's ability to perform useful work, and that impedes the mitochondrial performance leading to a gradual loss in their numbers making the type I muscles appear more like type II muscles. This leads to a greater propensity to muscle fatigue and spasm with a higher probability for injury and pain as a result of a reduced ability to presynaptically inhibit nociceptive reflexogenic afferents in the dorsal aspect of the spinal cord. This is a very common problem, and the brain suffers as a result.

15. Q: What is important to know about how these muscle types affect posture?

A: Any compromise in muscle function will complicate postural display, and vice versa. Since the postural display is of six different types—seven if you count normal, or balance—any one or a combination of these compensatory displays has its own rostral neuraxis concomitant and each has to do with the muscles involved. The four cerebellar postures—the flexion and extension synergies along with the right and left lateral bending—relate not only to the muscles on the ipsilateral side of the body but also to the function or adaptation of mitochondrial performance in those muscles. Remember, centerline structures relate to centerline nuclei. Any breakdown of the centerline stability affects the centerline brain, and that carries autonomic concomitants. The two thalamic postures also relate to the cerebellum but in this case the cerebellum has a secondary involvement. Because of their more rostral position, the thalamic postures—i.e., pyramidal displays—have increased complication. Each of these postures requires its own address unique to the patient's individuality.

ABOUT DR. ALLEN

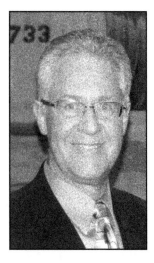

Dr. Michael Allen is an internationally recognized functional neurology teacher and also the author of the book, *What Your Brain Might Say if It Could Speak*, for the general public to better understand how to develop and keep a healthy brain, as well as several other professional papers.

Neurology has always been Dr. Allen's forté. His professional education includes graduating with honors from the Los Angeles College of Chiropractic in 1977. Since then he has become a Diplomate of the International Board of Applied Kinesiology (DIBAK), and the American Academy of Pain Management (DAAPM). He learned clinical neurology from Frederick Carrick, DC, PhD, founder of the Carrick Institute for Graduate Studies. Subsequently, Dr. Allen received Diplomate status from the American Board of Chiropractic Neurology (DABCN), and a Fellowship from the American College of Functional Neurology (FACFN). He is a member of the International College of Applied Kinesiology (ICAK), the Arizona Naturopathic Medical Association (AzNMA), and the German Medical Society for Applied Kinesiology (DAGAK, Hon.). He is a past member of the International Chiropractic Knights of the Round Table (1983-2008).

Dr. Allen has served the American Chapter of the International College of Applied Kinesiology (ICAK-USA) for 17 years as its Vice-President, Secretary, and Member-at-Large to the International Council of the ICAK, and as the International Council's President and Vice-President, overseeing eighteen chapters worldwide; he has also served on the ICAK's International Board of Standards (IBS), and as the Neurology Consultant to the ICAK Board of Examiners.

Index

E

F

P

CPSIA information can be obtained
at www.ICGtesting.com
Printed in the USA
FSHW04n0110210418
47115FS